Tuscarora Heroes

The War of 1812 British Attack on Lewiston, New York December 19, 1813

by Lee Simonson

Published by
Historical Association of Lewiston, Inc.
PO Box 43, Lewiston, New York 14092
716-754-4214

Fifth edition: August 2012
copyright 2010

ISBN: 978-0-557-31000-5

Cover art by Cindy Sanchez

"Shocking beyond description."

I never witnessed such a scene before and hope I shall not again.
 -- Charles Askin, Canadian citizen, 1813

They were stripped, scalped and had their hearts torn out."
 -- Baltimore Weekly Register, Jan. 29, 1813

The British entered the house at Lewistown in which the sick soliders and wounded lay, and not withstanding all the entreaties, shrieks and cries of the helpless soliders, not a life was spared, and it is reported that the houses were all burned before they were all dead.
 -- Niles Weekly Register, Dec. 24, 1814

The sight we witnessed was shocking beyond description. Our neighbors were seen lying dead in the fields and roads, some horribly cut and mangled with tomahawks, others eaten by the hogs, which were probably left for that purpose, as they were the only animals found alive.
 -- Portion of a Letter to the Editor from the
   Albany Argus, dated Buffalo, Dec. 26, 1813

The most savage cruelty was fiendishly enacted upon such as were unable to escape. The sequel was but another scene of distress and affliction, transpiring in bloody tragedy.
 -- Chipman P. Turner, Dark Days on the
   Frontier of Western New York, 1879

The citizens about Lewiston escaped by the Ridge Road, all going the one road on foot -- old and young, men, women, and children flying from their beds, some not more than half dressed, without shoes or stockings, together with men on horseback, wagons, carts, sleighs and sleds overturning and crushing each other, stimulated by the horrid yells of the 900 savages on the pursuit, which lasted eight miles, formed a scene awful and terrific in the extreme.
 -- Jonas Harrison, Lewiston resident
   Dec. 24, 1813

Lewiston was sacked, plundered, and destroyed – made a perfect desolation. Free course was given to the blood-thirsty Indians, and many innocent persons were butchered, and survivors were made to fly in terror through the deep snow to some forest shelter or remote cabin of a settler far beyond the invaders' track.
 -- Benson Lossing, Pictorial Field Book of the War of 1812, 1869

"Tuscaroras to the rescue..."

Bravery brought a company of armed Tuscaroras to the rescue, led by war-chief orator Longboard, Col. Johnson, Ovid and Littlegreen. They had heard the alarm and seen the torch, and fired a single volley which sufficiently surprised (the British and Mohawk natives) to cause a retreat and delay that furnished the inhabitants a few lucky minutes to escape from the blow of the tomahawk and thrust of the fatal knife.
-- Chipman P. Turner, Dark Days on the
Frontier of Western New York, 1879

It should be mentioned to the credit of a small band of Tuscarora Indians, that they effectually aided the flight of the citizens of Lewiston.
-- O. Turner, Pioneer History of WNY, 1850

Tuscaroras stood their ground long enough to allow the rest of the American force to escape. While the main body of Tuscaroras held their position, three warriors moved past the western tribesmen's flank, blew a horn, and fooled their enemies into thinking they were being surrounded.
-- Carl Benn, The Iroquois in the War of 1812, 1998

The Tuscarora Indians bravely repulsed a party of the enemy.
-- National Intelligencer, Washington DC, January 4, 1814

The overwhelming massacre was prevented by the appearance of Chief Longboard and his company. Their war whoop caused the attacking force to take at once to flight.
-- New York Times, April 8, 1883

It is evident that the timely intervention of the Tuscarora Indians, saved great slaughter of men, women and children among the white people. In every instance when the United States was in trouble, the Tuscaroras were ever ready to sacrifice their blood upon the American altar.
-- Tuscarora Chief Elias Johnson, 1888

CONTENTS

PART 1
Summary of the Attack and Rescue of
Lewiston Citizens by the Tuscarora Heroes

PART 2
Compilation of Primary Source and Reference Material

ONE COLD WINTER MORNING

In the annals of local and regional history, no event has caused more despair and torment than what occurred in Lewiston, New York, on the morning of December 19, 1813.

Even though it was just one morning during a war that lasted a thousand days, what happened was significant. It was the first wave of destruction that would eventually see Western New York in ashes, local residents killed, and local families torn apart.

Lewiston residents found themselves engulfed in a horrifying experience as they were attacked in their own homes by an overpowering enemy force that had no qualms about destroying civilian life or property.

To be sure, this is not a children's book, and there are graphic events that took place that morning that you will find upsetting.

The first part of this book provides an overview -- a quick summary of the attack and the events that led up to it.

The second part is a compilation of excerpts from various primary and reference sources that focus on the attack for those who are interested in reading the first hand details, without rewriting or filtered interpretation.

It is a bittersweet story.

On one hand, the founders of our Lewiston, New York, community were subjected to unimaginable horrors. Estimates of the number of civilians killed in the attack range from "some" to 46, with most in the dozen range. True figures will never be known, because records were destroyed, some families didn't move back to the area, and an undeterminable number of bodies perished within the burning homes and buildings.

In contrast to the tragedy, the long friendship with our Tuscarora neighbors manifested itself in a display of bravery and sacrifice that has never been duplicated.

Against all odds, the Tuscarora men stood by us that morning and put themselves in harm's way to protect us from the vicious attack. They served the American cause with distinction.

What I find bothersome is when Tuscarora Chief Elias Johnson wrote his History of the Tuscarora Indians in 1881, and reflected on the heroic efforts of his nation on behalf of the people of Lewiston. He expressed some resignation by saying, "but who cares anything about that?"

Mr. Johnson's feelings are understandable considering that in 1881 Native Americans were still enduring persecution and degradation by the United States government.

However, today in 2010, Lewiston citizens are finally understanding what happened on that cold winter morning, and want to let the world know that we do care!

That is why the Historical Association of Lewiston has published this book, and is planning to construct a large scale bronze monument -- aptly named, Tuscarora Heroes -- that will be unveiled on the 200th Anniversary of the attack. It will be a gift of thanksgiving to the Tuscaroras.

It will proudly stand for hundreds of years and will remind everyone, especially the citizens of Lewiston, about the courage and sacrifice the Tuscaroras made to protect our lives. It will also serve to let everyone know that we are privileged and honored to call the Tuscaroras our neighbors and friends.

We are indeed a grateful community.

Lee Simonson, Volunteer
Historical Association of Lewiston, Inc.
March 30, 2010

PART 1

Summary of the Attack and Rescue of Lewiston Citizens by the Tuscarora Heroes

LEWISTON'S NAMESAKE

No one could ever question the patriotism of Morgan Lewis.

Born to the privileged class in New York City, Lewis was never afraid to risk his life and property for the cause of freedom. His father was one of the signers of the Declaration of Independence and despite his social standing, he didn't hesitate to interrupt his law studies at Princeton to join the Revolutionary cause and take up arms serving as an officer in George Washington's army.

Later, as a distinguished and popular lawyer, he served in the New York Legislature and was elected New York's Attorney General. He even defeated Vice President Aaron Burr to become Governor of New York State in 1804.

Respected and admired, Lewis was accustomed to approbation, and as a gesture of esteem by his colleagues, Lewiston was named after him during his term as Governor. It was flattering, but Lewiston was in the most remote part of the state -- at the furthest edge of the frontier.

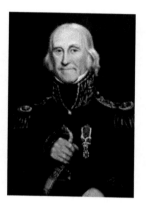

Lewiston was named after Gov. Morgan Lewis. He later served as a General in the War of 1812 on the Niagara Frontier. Did the decisions he made as General have anything to do with Lewiston's destruction during the war?

Several years later, Lewis would again take up arms, this time stationed on the Niagara Frontier as a General in the War of 1812. He would finally have a chance to visit the town that was named after him, and probably rode into Lewiston on horseback -- proud and confident that America could defend its frontier from the British-Canadian enemy.

However, through a strange set of circumstances, Lewis would be part of some fateful decisions that would have an impact on Lewiston's future as the War of 1812 dragged on -- decisions that would prove costly to Lewiston lives and property.

"TO MY UTTER ASTONISHMENT"

Months before Morgan Lewis arrived on the Niagara Frontier, blood was already being spilled.

The first major battle of the War of 1812 took place in Lewiston, where nearly half of the entire United States Army was stationed -- thousands of soldiers and state militia camped out along Center Street, the countryside, and near the river, waiting to invade and strike a crippling blow to Canada, which was a British colony at the time.

The War of 1812 was called the "Second American Revolution" and the War Hawks in the U.S. Congress were clamoring to chase British soldiers and influence out of the North American continent altogether.

The Americans had every advantage and significantly outnumbered the British. The troops were in high spirits and couldn't wait to engage the enemy. American General, Stephen Van Rensselaer, had a hard time holding them back.

Finally, in the early morning hours of October 13, 1812, the Americans took to the boats and the invasion began. The target -- Queenston, just across the Niagara River from Lewiston.

By late morning, the Americans had not only killed the revered British General Isaac Brock but were taking significant pieces of ground. A young 26 year old Virginian, a Lieutenant Colonel named Winfield Scott, gallantly led the charge and took control of the commanding heights of Queenston, on top of the Niagara Escarpment on the Canadian side. This was the beginning of a distinguished career that would see Scott become the longest serving General in American history -- "Old Fuss and Feathers" -- and one of the ablest commanders of all time.

Could it be that easy? Would former President Thomas Jefferson's prediction come true -- that forcing the British out of Canada would be a "mere matter of marching"?

Not quite.

The British had a secret weapon that would stop the Americans in their tracks -- it had nothing to do with guns, cannons or ammunition. Amazingly, it was sound.

When the Americans heard the war cries and whoops of the Mohawk natives who joined the British in a counter attack, the tide turned instantly and dramatically. The American soldiers could contemplate being struck by a British bullet and honorably dying on the field of battle. But if there was one thing the soldiers could not fathom, it was being axed or scalped by a tomahawk.

Despite orders to stand and fight, many of the American fighters who had made it to the Canadian side began to run and hide.

Pleading with the American militia to cross the Niagara River to reinforce their brothers who had taken the Heights, Van Rensselaer reported:

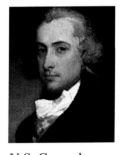

U.S. General Stephen Van Rensselaer was in charge of the American forces during the Battle of Queenston Heights in October 1812. He lost the battle when hundreds of American militia refused to cross the Niagara River to reinforce troops who had already taken the heights. They were afraid of being scalped.

"...to my utter astonishment, I found that at the very moment when complete victory was in our hands, the ardor of the unengaged troops had entirely subsided. I rode in all directions -- urged men by every consideration to pass over -- but in vain."[1]

Members of the militia,[2] still in Lewiston, began deserting in droves, or just stood there. The farmers and tradesmen who composed the militia suddenly became legal experts, quoting the state constitution stating that their duty was to defend the United States, not

---

[1] Letter from Van Rensselaer to his superior, Maj. Gen. Henry Dearborn, written the day after the battle. Reproduced on the Front Page of the New York Herald, Wednesday, November 4, 1812

[2] The militia was composed of ordinary citizens (not professional soldiers) who were called to take up arms during times of emergencies.

invade another country. Van Rensselaer couldn't even persuade his men to cross the river to rescue the soldiers who were pinned against the river's edge.

With no help, and no escape, Colonel Scott was forced to surrender and was taken prisoner along with 1000 other soldiers.

It was a crushing defeat for the Americans who were psychologically beaten and scared into raising the white flag[1] by a much smaller British force.

---

[1] Elting, John R., Amateurs to Arms: A military history of the War of 1812: "With no boats arriving to evacuate his men and with the Mohawks furious over the deaths of two chiefs, Scott feared a massacre and surrendered to the British. Even so, the first two officers who tried to surrender were killed by Indians, and after Scott had personally waved a white flag (actually Lt. Totten's white scarf), excited Indians continued to fire from the heights into the crowd of Americans on the river bank below for several minutes."

"I SHALL BAG THEIR WHOLE FORCE"

Six months after the defeat at Queenston, the Americans regrouped and wanted to take a second shot at invading Canada just across the Niagara River.

Meanwhile, Colonel Scott had been released in a prisoner exchange with the British and became the chief of staff for the American commander, General Henry Dearborn -- Dearborn, Michigan's namesake -- who was in charge of the military operations from the Niagara River to the New England Coast.

General Morgan Lewis, the connected politician, arrived on the scene and was placed second in command under Dearborn, mostly because of his personal friendship with President Madison and because he was the brother-in-law of the Secretary of War.

Dearborn had no respect for Lewis, calling him "totally destitute of any practical qualifications." On the other hand, Lewis saw Dearborn in terrible health, unable to make clear decisions, and with a military track record that was less than stellar. Dearborn knew of his unpopularity and even offered to resign months earlier.

But Dearborn and Lewis didn't have a monopoly on distrust. Strife among the American officers was rampant throughout the ranks. So much so that several of them challenged each other to duels. Who was the army fighting -- the British or themselves? In Washington, D.C., the army's inspector general complained about the quarrels, jealousies and plots within the Niagara campaign.

Despite the personal animosities, the Americans executed an almost perfect plan for the attack on Canada. The assault began with cannon fire from Ft. Niagara and schooners in the Niagara River, bombarding the British held Ft. George. Red hot cannon balls that had been put in furnaces and quickly loaded and shot, caused several buildings in Ft. George to catch fire.

On May 27, 1813, after the British defenses at the Fort had been badly compromised, the Americans launched a massive early morning assault by sea. Ft. George was surrounded, and the British General, John Vincent, realized he'd be forced to make a quick exit if he ever wanted to fight another day. He ordered the retreat, and Colonel Scott who led the amphibious assault was hot on his trail, hoping to crush and put a final stake in the fleeing British.

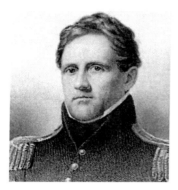

U.S. Colonel Winfield Scott was about to overtake the fleeing British enemy when he was stopped in his tracks. When he received his first order to stop his pursuit, he ignored it and kept going. Finally, after receiving his second order from Gen. Morgan Lewis, he relented and headed back. He was angry and resentful that he couldn't finish the job. Meanwhile, the British regrouped and within a few months were able to counter attack and invade the United States, capturing Ft. Niagara and burning Lewiston and Western New York to ashes. Scott later became the longest serving General in U.S. military history.

Then, inexplicably, U.S. General Morgan Lewis made a fateful decision and sent messengers to Scott to tell him to break off the pursuit. Colonel Scott, was dismayed, exclaiming to the messengers, "Your general does not know I have the enemy within my power. In seventy minutes I shall bag their whole force."

Defiant, Scott ignored the directive and continued his plans to catch the British.

Once again, Lewis sent a second set of orders to Scott to abandon the chase as he watched the fleeing British disappear in the woods. Scott was beside himself, but relented and headed back to Ft. George.

Subsequently, Dearborn and Lewis blamed each other for letting the enemy escape. The American stop-and-go attempts to finish off the British were unsuccessful.

Ten days later on June 6, 1813, with a chance to regroup and organize, the outnumbered British used a cunning strategy, along with some good fortune, and were able to turn back the Americans at Stoney Creek, Ontario, during a surprise nighttime attack. It was a turning point in the war.

A couple of weeks later, Laura Secord, a Canadian homemaker, overheard American officers who were occupying her house in Queenston, Ontario, planning another attack. She nonchalantly excused herself the next morning, and walked 20 miles through the woods and swamps to alert the British of the pending assault. With the warning from Laura and other British First Nations natives, nearly all the American soldiers were taken prisoner at the Battle of Beaver Dams.

That was the end of the American advances in Canada and Laura Secord became a Canadian heroine and legend.[1]

The pendulum was now swinging in the other direction and it was Britain's turn to begin its counter offensive that would not only drive the Americans off Canadian soil, but would enable the British to invade the United States, capture Ft. Niagara without firing a shot, and burn Lewiston to the ground while innocent men, women and children were slaughtered.

History will always ask: Did the order by Gen. Morgan Lewis to Colonel Scott, to break off the pursuit of the fleeing British, give the British an opportunity to reorganize and strike back?

Did that fateful decision cause a chain of events that would allow the British to regain their footing and push back, only to see the Lewiston, Buffalo and Western New York later destroyed?

---

[1] Laura Secord was actually an American citizen who was born in Massachusetts, but moved with her family to Canada in 1795 when she was 20 years old. She married a British loyalist two years later.

REVENGE!

Several months after the Americans had lost the Battle of Stoney Creek, the remaining U.S. forces, now under the command of Gen. George McClure, had retreated to a small defensive perimeter in and around Ft. George on the Canadian side of the Niagara River.

The Americans had captured Ft. George, but it turned out to be small prize for their efforts. Could the Americans even keep it?

No, they couldn't.

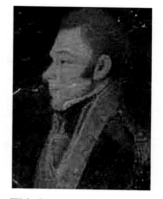

This is a rare image of U.S. Gen. George McClure who allowed the burning of the village of Newark (now Niagara on the Lake) Ontario. The British and the Canadians were enraged by the action against their civilians and used it as a battle cry to later burn Lewiston, and Western New York. Some historians even say that it was part of the reason the British burned the U.S. White House in 1814.

Most of the American soldiers in the area were reassigned to another hot spot -- namely, a planned attack on Montreal. Moreover, many of the militia enlistment terms were expiring. McClure was quickly losing men and that left the Americans extremely vulnerable to a British attack to take back Ft. George.

Half of McClure's force at Ft. George consisted of a group of men called Canadian Volunteers -- Canadian citizens who fought for the American side. The Americans considered them patriotic heroes -- the British looked down on them as outright traitors. The leader of the Volunteers was Joseph Willcocks, an elected official in Ontario, who was appointed an officer in the American army.

In late 1813, the noose was beginning to tighten and Gen. McClure got word the British were coming to get him. Without an adequate force, it would be suicide to stand and fight. McClure decided to abandon Ft. George and retreat a short distance across the Niagara River to Ft. Niagara on the American side.

What had been won by the Americans in a hard fought invasion was now being handed back to the British without even a fist fight.

On December 10, 1813, Gen. McClure allowed Joseph Willcocks[1] and his men to burn the Town of Newark (today's Niagara-on-the-Lake), which surrounded Ft. George in effort to deny the arriving British troops and their native allies shelter and supplies. With only a few hours of warning, scores of residents, including women and children, were driven into the snow without provisions. One historical account was written:

> In forcing the inhabitants -- mostly women and children (since the men were away in the army) -- out into the snow and bitter cold of a mid-December night, McClure was presumably hoping to deny the shelter of the village to the British forces who would now occupy the west side of the river.

> But it was a most ill-advised act and one subsequently disavowed by the American government. Ironically, the British forces, who had begun to advance on the frontier a few days earlier, came on so rapidly when they heard of the plundering that the American troops failed to

---

[1] Canadian Joseph Willcocks joined the American side in July 1813, and served as an officer. On September 4, 1814, he participated and led a charge at the Siege of Fort Erie. He was fatally shot in the chest. At first, his body was buried in "the circle or open square" in Buffalo, and then reburied in a mass grave at Forest Lawn Cemetery in the 1830s. One commentator stated, "Willcocks lies in an unmarked grave, ignored by the country he fought against and forgotten by the country he fought for."

destroy Fort George in their haste to cross the
river.[1]

McClure claimed he was following written orders,[2] but
his superiors denied it. Defending McClure, his officers stated
that the situation was handled humanely and that the residents
received plenty of time to evacuate and had the option of being
given food and shelter.[3] However, McClure was later fired by
the Secretary of War.

The debate will continue for centuries, but one thing
is clear -- the burning of Newark turned into a lightning rod
and infuriated the British, along with many Canadian citizens
who were still, at that point, indifferent and apathetic about
the War.

Jeopardizing the safety and lives of innocent civilians
was more than they could bear and the burning of Newark
was a turning point in galvanizing popular support in Canada
against the United States.

---

[1] Niagara Land: the First 200 Years, reprint of a series of essays
published in Sunday, the Courier Express Magazine, 1976.

[2] This was the exact order U.S. Gen. McClure received from the
Secretary of War in Washington, D.C, written on Oct. 4, 1813, regarding
the burning of Newark:

Sir: Understanding that the defense of the post committed to your
charge may render it proper to destroy the Town of Newark, you are
hereby directed to apprise its inhabitants of this circumstance and to
invite them to remove themselves and their effects to some place of
greater safety.

[3] Buffalo Gazette, Dec. 21, 1813, Letter to the Editor, signed by U.S.
Captain John Rogers, Brig. Major John Wilson, Lt. Donald Fraser:
"Twelve hours notice was given to the few inhabitants that remained to
secure their household property and every measure that could be taken to
alleviate their situation was done; three or four houses were left for those
that chose to remain; others who might wish to go across the river (to the
American side) the General ordered rations and quarters be provided
for."

Canada's respected historian, Pierre Burton, in his book, Flames Across the Border, wrote:

> In the hearts of the homeless and the soldiers there is one common emotion: a desire for retaliation. The senseless burning of Newark will send an echo down the corridors of history, for it is this act, much more than the accidental firing of the legislature at York, that provokes a succession of incendiary raids that will not end until the city of Washington itself is in flames.

Inflamed emotions were focused on only one thing now -- revenge!

FIRST PHASE: CAPTURE OF FORT NIAGARA

The British commanders began making plans immediately to vindicate the destruction of Newark. They decided to invade the United States. The attack would happen in two phases.

The first phase would be done in the middle of the night with the objective to capture Ft. Niagara on the American side.

The second phase would involve a large force of British soldiers and allied natives, primarily Mohawks, who would secure weapons in Lewiston that were thought to pose a threat to Queenston.

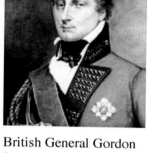

British General Gordon Drummond was the top commander of the British-Canadian forces on the Niagara Frontier.

The British knew that employing the First Nations natives could prove to be trouble and they could plainly see the handwriting on the wall.[1] They knew the savagery the Mohawks were capable of, and prior

---

[1] Two days before the British Attack on Lewiston, British Lt. Col. Harvey wrote to Col. Matthew Elliott, who was in charge of the native allies, with these orders from British Gen. Drummond:

"Sir - Lt. Gen. Drummond, having determined to avail himself of the services of his brethren and allies, the Western Indians, in an attack on the enemy's territory and fortress on the opposite shore, I have received His Honour's direction to request *you will assemble the several chieftains of those nations and will impress upon them in the strongest manner the expediency of abstaining from plunder and all acts of violence or outrage on the persons of women, children and unarmed men, and in the case of prisoners taken in arms.* The Lt. Gen. would willingly indulge the hope that, in conformity with the practice of their white brethren, the Western Indians will take a pride in showing their clemency and forbearance. Indeed, I am commanded by the Lt. Gen. that it is only upon giving their promise and assurance of observing his wishes on this head that he can consent to employ them on the service above alluded to." (Canadian Archives, C, 681, p. 260-1)

to the attack they went out of their way to admonish the war chiefs to show restraint and "abstain from plunder and all acts of violence or outrage on the persons of women, children and unarmed men."

But could the British control the Mohawks and other natives? Could the chiefs control their own men? Doubt lingered but the commanders had bigger issues to deal with at that moment.

Under the cover of darkness, late in the evening of December 18, 1813, the British began their methodical and calculated advance on Ft. Niagara.

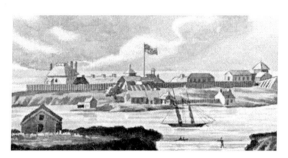

Armed with axes, scaling ladders and bayonets, over 500 British soldiers boarded their boats and quietly landed on the American shore about 3 miles south of Ft. Niagara. They silently walked toward the Fort, capturing American guards along the way -- one of whom was forced to give up the Fort's password for entry. When the British came to the Fort's gate, they confused a sentry long enough to storm past the defenders and rush in.

After giving up Fort George on the British-Canadian side of the Niagara River, the Americans lost Fort Niagara (above) in a surprise nighttime attack. Hardly a shot was fired. A few hours later, the British began the second phase of their assault on Lewiston.

The Fort's commander was at home a couple of miles away, and the American soldiers present were sleeping, drinking, or playing cards. Overwhelmed by the British, who came out of nowhere, the last minute American defense was futile. Dozens of Americans were killed by the bayonet in a most "horrid slaughter." [1] The others in the fort became instant prisoners -- outwitted, outfoxed and outmaneuvered.

---

[1] U.S. Gen. McClure letter to U.S. Secretary of War, Dec. 22, 1813

Historians wouldn't even call it a "battle" -- it is referred to as the "capture of Ft. Niagara."

The fort's huge 22 feet high x 28 feet wide American flag -- with 15 stars and 15 stripes -- considered the "older sister" of the Star Spangled Banner, was confiscated and taken as a war prize. It was sent to England and "laid at the feet of His Royal Highness and the Prince Regent" and later given to Gen. Gordon Drummond who was the top British commander during the Ft. Niagara siege.[1]

Handing over Ft. George to the British was one thing, but the British had just taken control of Ft. Niagara without firing a shot and were now on American soil -- firmly in command of Western New York's primary military fortress.

That would have been bad enough for the Americans, but the British had only begun to exact their revenge.

General Drummond had successfully captured Fort Niagara, and now the stage was set to execute his next plan. In a letter to his superior, Sir George Prevost, Drummond outlined his intentions the day before the attack:

> St. David's, December 18, 1813
> Major General Riall will follow immediately with the reserves and the Indians (under Col. Elliott) to act in support of Colonel Murray as circumstances may demand, independent of which I propose that an attack shall be made

---

[1] Ft. Niagara purchased the historic flag from the Drummond family in 1993 and restored it. It is now on display at Ft. Niagara in a special display case. Major George Armistead, from Virginia, was stationed at Ft. Niagara in 1813. Major Armistead loved big flags but he didn't like the cold weather here, so he asked for a transfer. On June 27, 1813, Major Armistead was happily reassigned to command Ft. McHenry in Baltimore, Maryland, where he ordered "a flag so large that the British would have no difficulty in seeing it from a distance." It was this 42' x 30' 15-star, 15-stripe flag, that gave inspiration to the defenders of Baltimore and inspired the national anthem. Ever since, the former Fort Niagara officer has been known as the "Guardian of the Star-Spangled Banner" which is now on display at the Smithsonian Institution.

upon Lewiston for the purposes of destroying
some works which the enemy have been
throwing up at that place with the avowed
intention of destroying from thence the town
of Queenston.

What happened next would change the course of the entire
war. While the British wanted to "destroy some works" in
Lewiston, the tactics the British employed would mimic today's
"shock and awe" campaigns -- a show of dominance so strong and
striking that it would send shock waves from here to Washington,
D.C.

Unfortunately for the civilians living in Lewiston, they
would find themselves not in the middle of the fight -- but on the
front line!

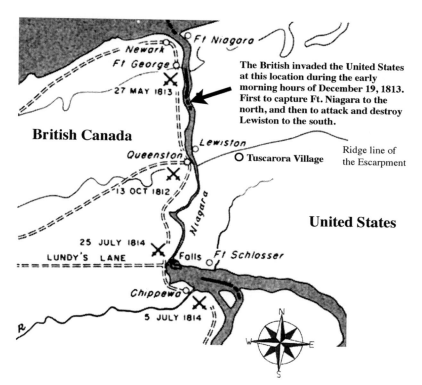

The British invaded the United States at this location during the early morning hours of December 19, 1813. First to capture Ft. Niagara to the north, and then to attack and destroy Lewiston to the south.

War of 1812 Map of the Lower Niagara River, including locations of major battles and dates.

SECOND PHASE: DESTROY LEWISTON

After the British had taken control of Fort Niagara at 5am on December 19, 1813, it was time for the second phase of the attack to begin.

It was Sunday morning, less than a week before Christmas. A canon was fired from Ft. Niagara. It was a signal to hundreds of British soldiers and their First Nations allies, waiting a few miles south, that the fort was securely in British hands and they could begin their retaliatory mission.

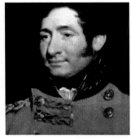

British General Riall was in command of the second phase which consisted of the 1st Royal Scots, the 41st Regiment (2nd Battalion) and hundreds of Mohawk natives -- a huge force.

They landed near today's Stella Niagara and began the vicious assault by heading south on River Road -- Lewiston was first on the agenda for retaliation. While the British command intended to "dislodge" any military batteries in Lewiston that posed a threat to them, the raid turned into much more -- it could only be characterized as a hellish conflagration of property and the bloody massacre of innocent lives.

British General Phineas Riall was in charge of the merciless force invading Lewiston. Despite orders to the contrary, the native allies of the British committed atrocities upon the Lewiston residents. Riall later went on to burn Buffalo. Western New York was in smoldering ruins.

The locals would easily admit that they could understand if the British wanted to burn Lewiston to the ground -- it would be an eye-for-an-eye and in measure with the burning of Newark. But what happened turned into much more. While the citizens of Newark were forced from their homes, the citizens of Lewiston were about to bleed. In both cases, military leaders let it happen.

Meanwhile, the local Tuscarora natives were on alert. For nearly a hundred years, they had established a long and friendly relationship with their Lewiston neighbors.

They had settled in Lewiston in the early 1700s, after being driven out of the Carolinas by the British. In one battle, nearly a thousand Tuscaroras were killed or captured.[1] They never forgot what the British had done to them and it was a compelling reason for their decision to side with the Americans, against the British, in both the Revolution and the War of 1812.

However, the Mohawks, their Iroquois[2] brothers, were strong allies of the British.

Ever since the British had taken back Ft. George several days before, tensions between the two sides of the Niagara River were high, and McClure had Canadian informants who warned of a British invasion.[3]

Suspecting the British would make a move against the United States, Tuscarora men remained vigilant atop the Escarpment. It was during the pre-dawn hours of December 19, 1813, when they first saw faint lights cross the river, presumably

---

[1] The Tuscarora War at Ft. Neoheroka, North Carolina, March 1713. The British and their native allies burned the fort and hundreds of Tuscarora men, women and children perished in the blaze. Almost two hundred more were killed outside of the fort and approximately four hundred Tuscaroras were taken captive and sold into slavery. The defeat of the Tuscaroras, once the most powerful native nation in the Carolinas, allowed the British to open up the frontier in the Carolinas to further expansion by European settlers. The survivors moved north and settled near Lewiston, becoming the sixth nation of the Iroquois Confederacy.

[2] The Village of Lewiston has named streets after the six nations of the Iroquois. Paralleling Center Street to the south are Cayuga, Seneca and Tuscarora Streets; and paralleling Center Street to the North are Onondaga, Oneida and Mohawk Streets.

[3] See page 120 for U.S. Gen. McClure's address warning that the British were going to attack on the night of Dec. 19th. The British actually attacked on the night of the 18th, the same day McClure penned his warning.

the lanterns from the British boats transporting the soldiers and native allies.

Under the command of their Tuscarora leader, Sachem Chief Solomon Longboard, two scouts were dispatched to see what was going on first hand, one being Jacob Taylor, better known as Colonel Jacobs.

The scouts reported that a massive British invasion was underway, including hundreds of British natives, composed mostly of Mohawks.

The Tuscaroras realized what was about to happen and scrambled to get the warning out to the Lewistonians, while mustering the men in their own village above the Escarpment to evacuate their women and children, and take up arms to -- somehow, someway -- fend off the attack.

But some families did not get the word in time.

The approaching enemy force was a juggernaut -- close to 1000 strong -- so imposing that the Lewistonians could do only one thing, and that was run for their lives!

One account summarized:

> The attack upon the village was after the Indian
> fashion, a sudden surprise. There was little
> warning; the Indians preceding for a few
> minutes, a detachment of British soldiers,
> swarmed out of the woods, and commenced an
> indiscriminate shooting down of flying citizens,
> plundering and burning.[1]

One of the first homes hit was the Alexander Millar family of "Mudball Hero" fame, living on a farm just north of the village on Lower River Road.

They heard the soldiers and natives and saw the lit torches fast approaching. Mrs. Millar and the younger children quickly hopped on a sleigh and headed out toward Ridge Road as fast as

---

[1] Turner, Pioneer History of the Holland Land Purchase, 1850

they could. Meanwhile, Mr. Millar and his teenage son Alexander, Jr.,[1] made the mistake of using precious time to protect the livestock. Fortunately, they weren't killed, but the delay cost them months of incalculable misery in a Montreal prison.

Other families didn't waste any time in fleeing. The Spaulding family was just sitting down for breakfast. Seconds later, they found themselves gathering the food in a tablecloth and running as fast as they could.

The exodus produced a panic never before seen in this area. With whatever clothes they had on their back, the local settlers were running through the snow and mud, in some instances in their bare feet. Parents were putting their children on passing carts, sleds or horse drawn wagons, praying they would have a better chance of escaping than remaining on foot. Scared families became separated and residents could only hope that somehow their lives would be spared.

The local physician, the beloved Dr. Joseph Alvord, who was disabled himself, jumped on his horse and started his hurried ride out of town. But it was too late. He was shot down and then tomahawked.[2] When he was found, his fingers were slit down to the wrists with hatchets -- inflicted upon him while he was holding his hands up to protect himself, or to ask for mercy.

And that was just the beginning.

---

[1] Before the outbreak of the war, at the height of international tensions between Canada and the U.S, some local Lewiston boys, including ringleader Alexander Millar, Jr., made a crude homemade cannon, and fired large mudballs at a passing British warship on the Niagara River. The British thought they were under attack and headed back down the river immediately, only later to find out that they had been spooked by the young pranksters.

[2] Dr. Alvord was shot down in front of his home at 6th and Center Streets.

Despite the British authority's admonishment before the attack, the rank and file Mohawk natives never heard the orders, or just simply ignored them and were intent on conducting a rampant killing spree. Even the top British Lt. General Gordon Drummond, later bemoaned:

> The Indians who advanced with Major Gen.
> Riall's force on the 19th had committed great
> excesses in consequence of intoxication.[1]

But when and where did the British natives become intoxicated? Some reports say that the Mohawks had imbibed on liquor left in the homes abandoned by the Lewiston citizens. Whether they drank before or during the attack remains open to speculation. Regardless, the situation turned ugly very quickly. Author Lewis Babcock wrote:

> Drummond exacted promises they would refrain
> from their usual savage practices. In the attack
> on Lewiston, they broke away from all restraint
> and used the tomahawk and scalping knife upon
> the dead, the wounded, and the unhurt,
> irrespective of sex or age.[2]

While British officers and soldiers wouldn't think about harming women and children in the heat of battle, the natives had no such custom or terms of engagement -- the enemy was the enemy, and that spelled doom to the small Lewiston population.

In some instances, the frenzied natives were able to remove themselves from the eyes of the British officers, freeing themselves to inflict carnage at will. If the British had not given the natives a license to commit "outrage," then the question will be asked for generations, "Why did the British enable them?"

---

[1] Drummond letter to Sir George Prevost, Dec. 22, 1813

[2] The War of 1812 on the Niagara Frontier, Babcock

As the blood thirsty attackers, who were supposedly under British control, set out to annihilate life and property, one heinous story stands out:

The Gillette family had moved to Lewiston from south of Albany to make a home in what was then the "far West." Life was good, and Solomon Gillette and his wife, Hepzipah, were raising five children: Miles, 19, Solomon's son from a previous marriage; and younger children Orville, Jervis, Alfred, and a year-old baby.

On that fateful morning, Solomon was returning home from Benjamin Barton's house on Center Street. Still unaware of the attack, he was suddenly taken prisoner by a group of British natives.[1] Fortunately, he wasn't harmed because there were British soldiers nearby. His son Miles, also unaware, was on the other side of the street and was also taken captive. But Miles fought back, grabbed a gun and shot one of the British natives. In turn, Miles was shot and scalped by the natives before his father's eyes.[2]

But even worse was what happened to Solomon's wife and four younger children at home.

Hepzipah had heard the strange distant boom earlier, not knowing it was the cannon shot at Ft. Niagara that signaled the attack. She and her son, Orville, 10, headed to the barn for an early morning milking of the cows. Suddenly they heard some confused noises and then "blood curdling yells cut the air."

Orville ran and hid as fast as he could, escaping the natives and eventually became lost outside of town. But Mrs. Gillette and

---

[1] Strangely, Solomon Gillette reported that some of his captors were actually white men in disguise, painted and dressed like British natives. Why would white Canadians feel the need to disguise themselves? Or, were the men in disguise actually Americans fighting for the British side who didn't want to be recognized? In another incident, reported in William Pool's History of Lewiston, New York, 1897, it is reported that a Lewiston woman killed two of the enemy after they had murdered her infant child. "After washing the soot off their faces she recognized two of her neighbors who were Tories (British supporters.)"

[2] Historian Chipman Turner says Miles was killed at 4th and Center Streets. However in a conflicting report, Clara Sisson Williams indicates that Miles was "killed by the Indians when Ft. Gray was taken."

the other younger children were cornered in the house. Three natives "threatened to brain the children and behaved like fiends in order to terrify their helpless captives."

Through an open door, she noticed a British officer down the road. If she could get to him, she thought, it might be a way to save her children from this real life nightmare. She bolted for the door while carrying Alfred, 4, and the baby. Following close behind was Jervis, 7. Her tormentors fired a gun and Jervis fell to the ground. A sad personal testimony revealed:

> One of the inhuman devils tore the scalp from
> his head before the breath left the body, and held
> it all reeking and bloody before the mother's
> eyes.[1]

The British officer witnessed the scene and ran over to make sure it wasn't repeated. But the horrors continued in other ways. Later, when her captors were distracted, Mrs. Gillette was able to escape, running out of town with her two remaining children, and spent two treacherous months, frostbitten and hungry, trying to reach her parent's home 270 miles away in Columbia County, with her two children.

She didn't know until a year later that her husband, Solomon, had survived and was released from a prison in Montreal, and that her 19 year old step-son, Miles, was killed the morning of the attack.

The other women and children who were not able to escape that terror filled morning were stripped of their clothing and taken across the river to Queenston as prisoners.[2]

---

[1] Clara Sisson Williams, Buffalo Historical Society, XXVI, Recalling Pioneer Days, 1922

[2] Robert Lee, Lewiston resident, deposition, Jan. 18, 1814, American State Papers, Military Affairs, Vol, I, p. 488, as published in Documentary History of the Campaigns Upon the Niagara Frontier in 1812-14, Vol. IX, by Cruikshank

The out of control rampage[1] was escalating so badly that the Mohawks started killing their allied British soldiers, and each other! One Canadian militia man wrote in his diary:

> We were obliged to keep a strong guard over the poor inhabitants -- men, women and children -- to prevent them from being killed by the Indians, one of whom was a young boy. Indeed, the Indians got so drunk that they did not know what they were about. They killed two of their own, and one solider of the 41 Regt. Mr. Caldwell, was shot through the thigh and young McDougall had his arm broken by another Indian who struck him with a tomahawk. Indians, regular British soldiers, and militia were plundering everything they could get a hold of.[2]

What small defense Lewiston had was composed of a small militia outpost under the direction of Major Bennett. Reports indicated that seven or eight men were killed defending Lewiston, including the sons of Captain Horatio Jones, the famous native

---

[1] A letter to the editor of Nile's Weekly Register from a gentleman on the Frontier said, "They killed at and near Lewiston eight or ten of the inhabitants, who, when found, were all scalped with the exception of one, whose head was cut off. Among the bodies was that of a boy ten or twelve years old, stripped and scalped." Benson Lossing, Pictorial Field Book of the War of 1812, published 1868, page 634.

[2] Charles Askin, Canadian militia, diary, Historical Collections of the Michigan Pioneer and Historical Society, Vol. XXXII, as published in Documentary History of the Campaigns Upon the Niagara Frontier in 1812-14, Vol. IX, by Cruikshank

interpreter.[1] But the soldiers knew they were outnumbered and outgunned and the small outfit saw many desert and run as soon as they "heard the yells of the Indians."[2] There was little resistance.

During the desperate escape out of Lewiston, minutes seemed like hours. Families did their best to extricate themselves from the inferno, bloody tomahawks and axes. Chipman Turner, a local historian summarized the travesty in the late 1800s:

> Consternation prevailed, beyond the control of the most cautious and deliberate. Men, woman and children were to be seen, in half clothed or almost naked condition, tramping in the snow, barefooted, creeping on their hands and knees, for concealment; turning from partly devoured meals, and hastily gathering the little that could be obtained, as reserve against the famishing hunger of themselves and children.[3]

In a horrifying scene, in an attempt to save their babies, mothers separated themselves from their own children, in hopes of retrieving them later:

---

[1] Brothers George W. and James W. Jones were killed after being taken prisoners. Their father, Horatio Jones, was appointed interpreter to the Iroquois Federation by George Washington. Publications of the Buffalo Historical Society, Vol. VI, states, "On attempting a division of spoil at Lewiston, the Indian warriors quarreled, worked themselves into a frenzy, and soon, beyond all restraint by the British, fell upon their prisoners. Here, within sight of the spot were Horatio Jones had come up on the crest of the mountain ridge on his memorable journey to Niagara, his two manly sons met the fate their father had so often narrowly escaped. They were put to death by the tomahawk, their bodies scalped and maltreated by the infuriated Mohawks."

[2] Charles Askin, Canadian militia, diary

[3] Chipman Turner, Pioneer Period of Western New York, 1918

At one time, five infant children, from their
mothers' breasts, were found upon the ox sled of
John Robinson, placed there by mothers anxious
to save their tender offspring. The mothers
adopted this as their only resort for the
children's protection, to save them from
slaughter or a life among the savages.[1]

One of Lewiston's residents and leading citizens, Jonas
Harrison,[2] was at the scene and gave this eye-witness account:

The citizens about Lewiston escaped by the
Ridge Road, all going the one road on foot --
old and young, men, women, and children flying
from their beds, some not more than half
dressed, without shoes or stockings, together
with men on horseback, wagons, carts, sleighs
and sleds overturning and crushing each other,
stimulated by the horrid yells of the 900 savages
on the pursuit, which lasted eight miles, formed
a scene awful and terrific in the extreme.

Every house in the village, save one, has been
burned; and the bodies of the massacred lie
about the streets, all of them scalped, many of
them disemboweled, some with their tongues
cut out, and all of them now being eaten by the
hogs.

Another Lewiston doctor, Willard Smith, was on foot and
was part of the tearful stampede out of town. He soon met up with
his friends, the Cookes, who lived a mile east of the village, along
the Ridge Road escape route.

---

[1] Chipman Turner, Pioneer Period of Western New York, 1918

[2] Jonas Harrison was the first Collector of Customs at Lewiston.

When the Cookes heard about the invasion, the women were sent ahead on horses. The elder, Lemuel Cooke, hitched his oxen and carried his ailing son, Lothrop Cooke,[1] to the sled. The father, Lothrop, and his brother, Bates, who was carrying a musket, headed out as fast as they could.

Dr. Smith asked Bates, "Is your gun loaded?" Bates said no. "Well, I have two cartridges, so load your gun with one, and I'll load mine with the other." The gift from Smith turned out to be providential.

Within minutes, when the Cookes were in the vicinity of what was known as Indian Hill, five British natives charged the sled on horseback. Their leader didn't have a hatchet -- he had a sword. And he rode up and took a mighty swing at Lothrop who was so weak he could hardly turn his head to avoid it. But the native missed and galloped a second time to make his kill.

As Lothrop looked up at the native's face -- thinking it would be the last thing he would ever see -- a shot rang out. His brother Bates[2] had used the one round of ammunition Dr. Smith had given him and took the shot he couldn't afford to miss. The

---

[1] Lothrop just had a leg amputated as result of an injury he sustained a year earlier fighting in the Battle of Queenston Heights and was very ill.

[2] Joshua Cooke, Souvenir History of Niagara County, 1902. The writer, Joshua, was the son of Bates Cooke, the man who shot the British native in the neck. Two years later in 1815, Bates became a lawyer and was admitted to the bar. Years later, Bates was elected to Congress as an Anti-Mason and later became New York State Comptroller, the only person from Lewiston who has ever attained statewide office. He is buried in the Village of Lewiston cemetery, next to the Presbyterian Church.

attacker[1] was hit square in the neck, fell off his horse[2], staggered and dropped dead.[3]

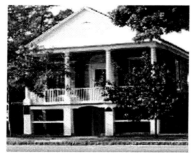

This building at 755 Center Street in Lewiston was built in 1820 by Bates Cooke who used it as his law office, replacing a building that had been burned down during the British attack in 1813. Bates and his family were run out of town during a harrowing experience in which he killed a British native while defending his disabled brother.

---

[1] Turner, Pioneer History of the Holland Land Purchase, 1850. "In the pocket of the dead Indian was a paper addressed to the Indian Agent at Niagara (Ontario) saying that the bearer was an 'Ottawa brave, worthy of being entrusted with any daring expedition.'"

[2] Margaret Robson, Under the Mountain, 1958. "The dead Indian's horse was found and used by the Cookes to help them reach safety. Bates Cooke had been a lawyer in Lewiston and after the war one of the first cases he handled was to determine the ownership of the horse he had taken. The horse had a U.S. Government brand on it and had belonged to the army until it had been captured by the British. Bates argued that since the horse had been captured by the enemy it belonged to anyone who should recapture it. He won title to the horse and sold it to get enough money to set himself up in a law office again (his old office and all of the law books had been burned in the attack.)"

[3] A handwritten letter detailing the Cooke's plight was discovered in September 2010. It is from Isaac C. Cooke, brother of Lothrop and Bates. You can find a transcription of the letter on page 142.

TUSCARORA HEROES

At that moment, the Tuscarora men swung into action.

The small force had run down the Escarpment from their village above the hill and had witnessed the Cookes plight from behind the cover of trees.

Conflicting reports indicate that the party of Tuscaroras was led by either Jacob Taylor, known affectionately to locals as Colonel Jacobs, and described as a "small, thin, wizened man, with the soul of a hero," [1] or by John Obediah. [2]

The Tuscaroras fired their muskets, and screamed a war whoop -- the first serious resistance the British or their native allies had seen or heard. Shocked by seeing their leader killed, and now being fired upon by the American natives, the remaining British natives galloped off and retreated into the woods.

While most of the American militia deserted and snuck out of Lewiston, the Tuscaroras not only stood strong, but ran into the fight in an effort to save their neighbors.

Strangely, when it came to holding back the enemy, it turned out that the Lewiston residents could only count on the brave Tuscaroras and the gallant efforts of Major Mallory, and a small force of about forty Canadian Volunteers[3] who were stationed in Niagara Falls and were able to temporarily slow a part of the British contingent who were attempting to advance south.

The Tuscaroras knew they were grossly outnumbered 30 to 1, so whatever they could do to thwart the attack and buy precious minutes, would have to be done quickly, carefully and shrewdly.

The Tuscaroras were not thinking about a counterattack. Their rescue mission was purely a defensive operation and the objective was to mitigate the catastrophe and facilitate the rapid evacuation of the town.

---

[1] Joshua Cooke, Souvenir History of Niagara County, 1902

[2] Chief Elias Johnson, History of the Tuscarora Indians, 1881

[3] Canadians who fought on the U.S. side during the War of 1812.

That meant a series of diversionary tactics would have to be employed. The object would be bluff the enemy and create an illusion of strength without getting anyone killed in the process.

No one knew the Escarpment and geography of the area better than the Tuscaroras and they used that knowledge to leverage their plan to save as many lives as they could.

Despite the Tuscarora's untenable situation of being outmanned and outgunned, it didn't stop them from executing a courageous and brilliant strategy within minutes.

The Tuscarora Chief, Solomon Longboard, directed the operation and sent some men to the top of the Escarpment, just above the Mohawks below. The men started blowing horns from several locations along the edge of the Escarpment cliff, giving the impression that there was a large unseen force of American natives ready to launch a counterattack from the heights.

At the same time, another group of Tuscarora men "rushed down the mountain with their war whoops as if a legion were coming down." [1] The sight and sound of the Tuscarora advances spooked the Mohawks who were still chasing the column of Lewiston citizens trying to escape. Unsure of what they were facing, and not wanting to run into a trap, the Mohawks stopped in their tracks and retreated about a mile and a half back to the Lewiston village where the main British force was stationed.

One story about their retreat involved a stand off between one Tuscarora and a British native, as related by Tuscarora Elias Johnson:

> Then one of the men (a British native) halted
> and aimed his gun at one of our men, John
> Obediah. Obediah aimed back, while Samuel
> Thompson got behind a large elm tree. In the
> meantime, John Obediah spoke to the stranger

---

[1] Elias Johnson, History of the Tuscaroras, 1881. This occurred on Ridge Road at the intersection of the old Indian Hill Road, which no longer exists. It is a little over a mile east of Creek Road (Rt. 18) and long time locals would know it as the place of the old ski slope on the Escarpment.

in all the different six languages of the Iroquois,
but did not get an answer. Finally the British
Indian retreated backwards, keeping aim as he
went, and all at once gave a spring and ran off.

While the Tuscarora plan was based primarily on bluff and
bluster, it was tremendously risky. Facing an enemy -- eye to eye
and gun to gun -- was proof of the fearlessness and tenacity of the
Tuscaroras at that critical moment. Had the true strength of the
Tuscaroras been realized, their fate would have been sealed.

When the last British native was seen running back to the
Lewiston village, enough time was gained to enable the safe
eastward passage of the fleeing citizens on Ridge Road who were
lucky enough to escape the onslaught. Elias Johnson wrote:

By this time, the train of white people had gone
quite a good ways in their flight: it is evident
that the timely intervention of the Tuscarora
Indians, saved great slaughter of men, women
and children among the white people.

The swift strategy and courage of the Tuscaroras bought
precious minutes by creating a wedge, or buffer zone, between the
attackers and the destitute citizens. However, the British and their
Mohawk allies had no intentions of stopping their pursuit
indefinitely.

The Mohawks were furious with the Tuscaroras for helping
the Lewiston residents, and there would be payback. Next stop for
the attackers: The Tuscarora village, atop the Lewiston
Escarpment.

Knowing there would be consequences for their actions,
and willing to make the sacrifice, the Tuscaroras had quickly
vacated their village and made sure their women and children were
safe. With most of the Tuscaroras defending the rear of the train of
sufferers on Ridge Road, the Tuscarora village was defenseless and
the Mohawks began indiscriminately burning their homes and
winter food supplies. It was complete devastation.

Realizing they had destroyed both Lewiston and the Tuscarora villages, the Mohawks gained a second wind and wanted to chase down the fleeing residents.

Ridge Road was the main road into and out of Lewiston. It was a dirt road and conditions were terrible. Lewiston citizens did their best to navigate the ruts, the mud, and the snow, as they traveled east as fast as they could. No one could predict when or if the invading force would strike again. The sufferers could only push on in hopes of freeing themselves from horrors they had just witnessed.

When they had gone about nine miles, some of the Lewiston men in the procession had arrived at a large log house[1] which was used an armory. As they were breaking open the powder kegs to set it on fire in an effort to prevent the British from

---

[1] Vernette Genter, former Town of Cambria Historian, The Evolution of Niagara County. "No one was spared until the marauders reached the vicinity of the intersection of what are now Baer and Church Roads (and Ridge Road), where residents had stored a supply of ammunition in a log schoolhouse. With the help of the friendly Tuscaroras from the Reservation, the settlers were able to repulse the raiders and send them scurrying back to Lewiston. As a result, Howell's Tavern, east of the schoolhouse, was spared, as was the Forsyth Tavern." Bear and Church Roads intersect Ridge Road (Rt. 104) nine miles east of the Village of Lewiston where the attack began. Assuming the attack on Lewiston began at approximately 7am, and the line of fleeing citizens were able to move at 2 miles per hour on Ridge Road, they would have arrived at the log house in Cambria approximately 11:30am on the morning of Dec. 19, 1813.

In another reference as to the location of the log house, Chipman Turner reports in 1879, "The rallying point was fixed at the two temporary arsenals, consisting of two log dwellings, that stood on the east and west corners, now owned by Amos B. Gallop (the original foundation is still visible) and Peter Oliphant, on the south ridge, half a mile west of Howell's creek (12 Mile Creek), near where the settlement in the county was first commenced by Philip Beach, in 1801. One of the buildings was used for a deposit of powder, the other for arms."

capturing any of the supplies, Tuscarora leader Solomon
Longboard arrived on the scene.

With the help of one of his men and interpreter, Colonel
Jacobs, Chief Longboard convinced the Lewiston men to save the
building and the powder and to keep advancing east, out of harm's
way. The Tuscaroras would take a stand.

Elias Johnson reported:

> When the British Indians came in sight, Mr.
> Longboard instructed his men to keep moving
> back and forth from the log house or armory, to
> a thicket in the rear of the house, for the purpose
> of making the enemy believe that there was a
> large force stationed there; the enemy halted and
> finally went back, and thus the armory was
> saved.

The Tuscaroras drew the line in the sand, and the residents
of Lewiston continued to migrate out of Niagara County, in many
instances on foot, to rebuild their shattered lives.

However, the destruction of Lewiston was only the first
stop for the British.

Two days later, on December 21, 1813, General Riall and
his British soldiers and natives went on to destroy Manchester
(now Niagara Falls, New York) and the small military outpost
there, Fort Schlosser. The British continued to scorch and burn
everything in their path until they reached Tonawanda Creek, now
North Tonawanda. The Americans had destroyed the bridge there
so the British couldn't pass over it. The British then retraced their
steps back to Canada and regrouped for a new nighttime attack.

In the early morning hours of December 30, 1813, the
British silently crossed the upper Niagara River and attacked
Buffalo at Black Rock. Despite warnings and a build up of
American troops, there was no stopping the British. They easily
defeated the Americans, many of whom had deserted, and burned
Buffalo to the ground, in the same fashion they had done to

54

Lewiston eleven days earlier -- again, in retaliation for the American burning of Newark.
Western New York was in ashes.

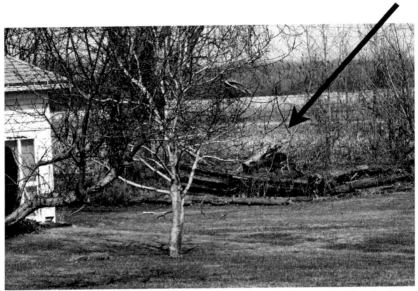

Photograph taken April 2011

Ruins of Log Cabin Where Tuscaroras Drew Line in the Sand

This photograph shows the ruins of what is believed to be the log cabin where the Tuscaroras took a stand and held back the enemy, after instructing the Lewiston survivors to continue their escape east on Ridge Road. The cabin is on private property that was originally owned by the Hillmans, and most recently owned by Eman and Mildred Maulis.

The cabin is located in the backyard of the family home on the north side of Ridge Road, about 2/10s of a mile east of today's Faery's Nursery. It had remained standing and intact until a tree branch fell into it several years ago, destroying the roof and most of the structure.

THE SUFFERERS

One writer called it "a winter of gloom and despondency." Historian Chipman Turner, quotes another commentator:

> A gloomy stillness brooded over the scene, so profound, that the gaunt wolf, usually stealthy and prowling, came out of his forest haunts at mid-day, and lapped the clotted snow, or snatched the dismembered limb of a human corpse that in haste and flight had been denied the right of sepulture.[1]

Those who were on the run and displaced were called "the sufferers" -- all caught in a panicked confusion, not knowing where they were going, or where they would find their next meal.

> On the road between Cayuga and LeRoy, a traveller met more than a hundred families in wagons, sleighs and sleds, and found the Tuscarora Indians encamped in the woods without shelter. The Governor of New York said, "The panic which these transactions have spread among the inhabitants is inconceivable. They are abandoning their possessions and flocking to the interior."[2]

Citizens who lived outside of the areas that were attacked and who were spared the hardships and atrocities, formed a committee to begin raising funds in a humanitarian effort to help the sufferers. It was called the Committee of Safety and Relief of Canandaigua. On January 8, 1814, the Committee received this heartbreaking report:

---

[1] sepulture: the act of placing in a sepulcher or tomb; burial.

[2] Cruickshank, Drummond's Winter Campaign, Second Edition

Niagara County, and that part of Genesee which lies west of Batavia are completely depopulated. All the settlements in a section of the country 40 miles square and which contained more than 12,000 souls are effectively broken up. These facts you are undoubtedly acquainted with; but the distresses they have produced, none but the eye-witness can thoroughly appreciate.

Our roads are filled with people, many of whom have been reduced from a state of competence and good prospects, to the last degree of want and sorrow.

The fugitives from Niagara County especially, were dispersed under circumstances of so much terror, that, in some cases, mothers find themselves wandering with strange children, and children are seen accompanied by (adults) who have no other sympathies with them than those of common sufferings.

Of the families thus separated, all the members can never meet again, in this life; for the same violence which has made them beggars, has forever deprived some of their heads, and others of their branches.[1]

Lt. Col. E. Cruikshank, a Canadian historian, observed:

The destruction of Niagara (Newark) had been avenged ten-fold, and the wretched inhabitants on both sides of the river had suffered in turn all the miseries that war could inflict.[2]

---

[1] Louis Babcock, The War of 1812 on the Niagara Frontier, 1927

[2] Cruickshank, Drummond's Winter Campaign, Second Edition

Thousands of dollars in private donations to help the sufferers poured in. The state and federal governments also appropriated money. New York State authorized $40,000 be given to the sufferers, and $5000 to the Tuscaroras for the tribe's losses. Another $5000 was given to Canadians who had taken refuge in New York State.[1]

While many citizens never returned to the area, some hearty souls came back to start their lives from scratch.

In Lewiston, many of the determined pioneers put the nightmare behind them and began to pick up the pieces to construct some of the finest structures that still exist today. As an example, the Frontier House was built in 1824 and was considered the finest hotel in the United States, west of the Hudson River.

The War of 1812 lasted nearly three years, and was finally settled in February of 1815. It was fought on land and sea -- from as far north as Montreal to as far south as New Orleans -- and many notable events took place including the burning of the White House, and the birth of America's national anthem, The Star Spangled Banner.

Who won the War of the 1812? Legally, the war was considered a tie.

Nonetheless, Canadians believe they won because they were successful in driving Americans off their soil and that they never became part of the United States.

Americans believe they won because the British stopped interfering in American affairs. With British influence gone, America was free to achieve Manifest Destiny and eventually expand to California, rather than be limited to 18 states. The United States went from being a country few took seriously to becoming a player with a seat at the international table.

---

[1] Louis Babcock, The War of 1812 on the Niagara Frontier, 1927. Historical details are sketchy on how these Canadians were identified. Most likely, they were families of the Canadian Volunteers who were a group of Canadians who sided with the Americans.

For Lewistonians, who were true frontier settlers at the time, the War also proved to be a turning point. Unimagined hardships and losses were confronted and overcome, and life began to return to normal as Lewiston became the "Gateway to the West" between 1815 and 1825.[1]

The War of 1812 taught the citizens of Lewiston a valuable lesson. While they will always view the attack with regret, they also learned that friendship and patriotism were more than just words.

They realized that when trouble was near, and lives were at stake, they could count on the heroic actions and deeds of their Tuscarora neighbors who bravely rescued them on that cold winter morning.

For that, Lewiston citizens will be forever grateful.

---

[1] Once the Erie Canal opened in 1825, most of the commerce shifted to Buffalo, and Lewiston's role on the trade routes was greatly diminished. However, Lewiston did become a major Great Lakes passenger port during the latter 19th and early 20th Centuries -- hosting up to 20,000 passengers a day. The invention of the automobile eventually put the passenger steamships out of business.

PART 2

Compilation of Primary Source and Reference Material

Orsamus Turner
Pioneer History of the Holland Purchase of Western New York
Published by Jewett, Thomas & Co., 1850

The force that landed at the Five Mile Meadows under Col Murray was about 500 -- they completed the landing before daybreak.

A party of Indians, leaving the main body, came up to Lewiston -- arriving about sunrise. There was stationed there but a small force under the command of Major Bennett, that retreated with the loss of six or seven men; among whom were two sons of Horatio Jones. The attack upon the village, was after the Indian fashion, a sudden surprise. There was little of warning; the Indians preceding for a few minutes, a detachment of British soldiers, swarmed out of the woods, and commenced an indiscriminate shooting down of flying citizens, plundering and burning. Among the slain in the attack on Lewiston was Dr. Alvord who has been mentioned as the early physician at Batavia. He was shot from his horse while endeavoring to make his retreat. Miles Gillette and a younger brother, sons of the early pioneer Solomon Gillette, Thomas Marsh, William Gardner, Tiffany and Finch.

That day, December 19th, the Ridge Road presented some of the harshest features of war and invasion. The inhabitants upon the frontier en masse were retreating eastward; men, women and children; the Tuscarora Indians having a prominent position in the flight.

The residents upon the Ridge that had not got the start of the main body fell in with it as it approached them. There was a small arsenal at the first four corners west of Howell's creek[1], a log building, containing a number of barrels of powder, several hundred stand of arms, and a quantity of fixed ammunition. Making a stand there, the more timid were for firing the magazine and continuing the retreat. The braver councils prevailed to a small extent. They made sufficient demonstrations to turn back a

---

[1] Near today's intersection of Ridge Road (Rt. 104) and Church Street, in the Town of Cambria.

few Indian scouts that had followed up the retreat to plunder such as fell in the rear.

The mass made no halt at the arsenal, but pushed on in an almost unbroken column until they arrived at Forsyth's where they divided, a part taking the Lewiston Road and seeking asylums in Genesee County, and over the river; and a part along the Ridge Road, and off from it in the new settlements of what is now Orleans and Monroe counties, and in what is now Wayne, and the north part of Ontario counties.

All kinds of vehicles were put in requisition. It was a motley throng, flying from the torch and the tomahawk of an invading foe, without hardly the show of a military organization to cover their retreat.

Almost the only resistance that the invaders encountered, was an attack upon Lewiston Heights, in their attempted advance to Niagara Falls, by Major Mallory and his small corps of Canadian volunteers who were stationed at Schlosser. They compelled them to retreat below the mountain, and afterwards contested the ground to Tonawanda, with a bravery that was the more creditable, as it was a rare article at that unfortunate period.

And it should be mentioned to the credit of a small band of Tuscarora Indians, that they effectually aided the flight of the citizens of Lewiston, by firing upon the Indian scouts that were following them up, from an ambush, upon the side of the mountain, near where the road from their village comes upon the Ridge. It helped to turn back the pursuers.

There are many interesting reminiscences connected with the attack upon Lewiston and the flight of its citizens, but a small portion of which can be given in this brief notice of the events of the war.

At the period of the invasion, Judge Lothrop Cooke, was an invalid, having had, but a short time previous, one of his legs amputated. He was laid upon an ox sled, and accompanied by his brother, the late Hon. Bates Cooke. When they had proceeded but a few miles upon the Ridge, a scout of five Indians overtook them, and ordered a halt. Bates Cooke seized a gun that was lying upon a sled directly behind them, fired, and shot one of the Indians through the neck. He fell from his horse, jumped upon his feet, and after running about fifteen rods, fell and died. Mr. Cooke, having no further means of defense, ran -- the Indians making two ineffectual shots at him in his retreat.

The firing of the guns brought some Tuscarora Indians to the spot, who fired upon the British Indians that remained, and compelled them to turn back. The sled with the invalid passing on in safety. In the pocket of the dead Indian was found a paper addressed to the Indian Agent at Niagara saying that the bearer was an "Ottawa brave worthy of being entrusted with any daring expedition."

There is a solitary grave upon the Ridge Road near the eastern extremity of Hopkin's Marsh.[1] It is that of a teamster whose name was Mead. He was conveying some household furniture from Lewiston in the morning of the invasion. An Indian overtook and shot him. This was the farthest advance that either the British or Indians made upon the Ridge Road.

---

[1] It is believed Hopkin's Marsh was located near the Lewiston-Cambria town line.

Mrs. Clara L. Sisson Williams[1]
An Experience of 1813
A True incident of the Niagara Frontier
Publications, Buffalo Historical Society
Recalling Pioneer Days, XXVI – 1922

The winter of 1813-14 is memorable in the history of Western New York for the whole Niagara Frontier was laid waste by the British regulars and their bloodthirsty Indian allies. Buffalo and other villages were burned and many settlers killed.

Those who escaped fled in terror through the deep snow to the sheltering forest, or to some lonely cabin in the wilderness.

The Gillette family lived at Lewiston on Niagara River seven miles below the falls. They had moved from Columbia County in the eastern part of the state to make a home in what was then the far West, the Holland Purchase.

There were four children in the family besides Miles, a youth of nineteen, who was the son of Mr. Solomon Gillette by a former marriage. Orville was a sturdy lad of ten; Jervis and Alfred were seven and four years of age respectively, and the baby was about a year old.

The evening of December 18, 1913 found Mrs. Gillette alone in the living-room of their comfortable log house. The short winter day had seemed long to her because of fear and anxiety, but at last darkness settled down over the snow-covered earth. The scattered cabins of the village were dimly outlined against the sky, and the roar of the mighty river sounded faintly in the distance.

Within was light and warmth from the great fireplace, which nearly filled one end of the room. The curtains were closely drawn over the small window with their diamond-shaped panes; and the doors were securely fastened. A supply of wood was neatly piled at one side of the "clean-winged hearth." Over the mantle, which held many small articles useful and ornamental,

---

[1] The writer of this true sketch is a granddaughter of Solomon Gillette of Lewiston. Her mother was born in Lewiston in 1817. Mrs. Williams resided in Batavia.

hung a pair of antlers. Ears of maize, hunks of dried venison and rings of dried pumpkin swung from the smoky ceiling. The bare floor was clean as hands could make it. A tall clock, reaching from floor to ceiling occupied one corner and a small flax-wheel another. There were a few splint-bottomed chairs, a settle and a homemade table. The door opening into another room, where the children were sleeping stood ajar, that the mother might hear the slightest sound from within. It was a handsome face illuminated by the firelight, handsome notwithstanding its careworn expression; the features clear-cut and regular, the skin fair, while the hair and eyes were of jetty blackness.

Her knitting fell from her hands and a look came into the great black eyes, as in fancy she wandered back to her childhood's home of the banks of the Hudson, where her father and brothers tilled their fertile acres in quiet prosperity. Their life was very different from that of the frontier, even in times of peace. Now the contrast is stronger than ever.

The expressive face changed again as she thought of her husband and stepson, who were with a detachment of militia, under Maj. Bennett, stationed on Lewiston Heights. This battery was called Fort Gray. Fort Niagara was at Youngstown, seven miles further down the river.

An invasion was feared, and with good reason -- for the Americans had abandoned Fort George and retreated across Niagara River. Before doing so General McClure, the commanding officer, burned the village of Newark in order to prevent the enemy from using it as quarters for their troops during the winter. There was no necessity and no excuse for the destruction of this village, and it was speedily avenged by the enemy.

The hours passed slowly to the lonely woman, whose mind was too full of a nameless dread to allow her to seek repose. She dozed in her chair, now and then rising to replenish the fire.

Just as the first rays of dawn lighted the East a heavy booming sound, not unlike distant thunder, broke the stillness. She was unable to account for the sound at the time, but afterward knew that it was the signal that Fort Niagara had fallen. "A signal for the ear of Gen. Riall, who, with a detachment of British regulars and about 500 Indians, was waiting for it at Queenston. Riall immediately put his forces in motion, and crossed the Niagara to Lewiston, overpowered the small detachment of militia and took possession of the village."

Mrs. Gillette, thoroughly aroused by the report of the cannon, woke her eldest son, Orville, and soon after they went to the barn in the rear of the house to milk and fodder the cows and do the other chores. The younger children were left in the house.

After placing a generous supply of cornstalks in the mangers, the mother and son proceeded to milk "Brindle" and "Suky." The task was nearly done, when they heard a strange, confused noise from the direction of the river. They dropped the milk-pails and looked at each other in dismay. Bloodcurdling yells cut the air.

"Mother, let's run to the house," faltered the boy with blanched face.

There was not time to act on this suggestion. Three Indians, hideous in war-paint and feathers, were making directly for the open door of the stable. The savages lost no time in fruitless parley with their prisoners, but two of them immediately began to search the barn for plunder. Their companion found a pail partly filled with milk, which he drank with great relish. When at last the head emerged from behind the pail the boy was gone.

There happened to be a number of haystacks near the barn, and Orville, quickly seeing an opportunity to escape, ran from the stable, and dodged behind the nearest stack, and from one to another, keeping them between himself and the barn until he reached the last one. Then he ran toward the woods; ran as only a frightened boy can run.

Two of the Indians pursued him, but he had the head start and was out of range of their muskets. They soon gave up the chase and returned to the congenial work of sacking a burning the village.

The lad pressed on, sometimes running and sometimes walking. He gained a road leading into the interior and could make better headway than when in the tangled wood. After traveling three or four miles he came to a log cabin and stopped to warn the inmates of coming danger, but they had already fled with such valuables as they could carry.

Their untasted breakfast stood smoking on the hearth, and the hungry boy helped himself to the food.

As he stood by the fire munching a piece of corn bread he noticed that his tracks across the floor were bloody; and he found that his ankles were cut to the bone by the hard steely crust on the snow. His shoes were low and he had broken through the crust at every step.

He plodded on all day, occasionally passing the deserted home of a settler; and it was one of these houses that sheltered the weary, heartsick boy that night.

Late in the afternoon of the second day he arrived at a small settlement, and found a temporary home in the family of a kindhearted Methodist preacher, to whom he told his story.

Orville's mother and brothers were doomed to suffer more than he. When the two Indians started in pursuit of the son the remaining savage drove the mother before him to the house, which he soon ransacked. He found a demijohn of whisky, imbibed freely and seemed to like it exceedingly. At this juncture three more braves arrived, and in a few minutes all were quarreling over the "firewater."

They threatened to brain the children and behaved like fiends in order to terrify their helpless captives, and really appeared to enjoy the sport.

Mrs. Gillette held the two younger children in her arms and Jervis hung to her skirts. Through the open door she could see a British officer, in a gay uniform, farther down the street.

"If we could only get to him and put ourselves under his protection our lives would be spared," she reasoned.

She determined to make the attempt. And as the attention of her tormentors was just then given to the demijohn, she sprang through the doorway with the two children in her arms, followed closely by Jervis.

The Indians, maddened by drink, fired a volley at the fugitives. Little Jervis fell. One of the inhuman devils tore the scalp from the head before the breath left the body, and held it all reeking and bloody before the mother's eye.

The British officer saw the deed, and filled with anger at the wanton cruelty of the Indians, hurried to the spot in time to prevent their doing further mischief.

History informs us that "Lewiston was sacked, plundered and destroyed -- made a perfect desolation. Eight or ten of the inhabitants were killed and scalped, with the exception of one, whose head was cut off. Among the bodies was that of a boy seven or eight years old, stripped and scalped." This boy was Jervis Gillette.

For several days the heartbroken mother was a prisoner, suffering many indignities and hardships. But she escaped one dark stormy night while the Indian guard lay in a drunken sleep, and was miles away when her flight was discovered.

Her progress was necessarily slow, encumbered as she was by two little children. She was obliged to carry the baby. Alfred walked clinging tightly to his mother's hand. But he was only four years old, and soon became tired and began to cry. As often as this happened the poor woman was obliged to stop and rest, or else carry both children.

Homeless, friendless, penniless, distracted by grief -- behind her the relentless enemy and the ruins of her once happy home -- before her a thinly settled country covered deep by the snows of midwinter. What could she do? There was only one thing to do; she would go home to her father's house.

Words are inadequate to describe the sufferings of that journey, suffering from cold, hunger and weariness. Two hundred and seventy miles across the state over miserable roads she tramped, begging her way. Occasionally she rode a short distance on the ox-sled of some farmer.

Most of the people were kind when they had heard her sad story, and willingly gave food and shelter; and some added warm clothes, encouraging words, and even a little money. Others refused to believe her story and gave her only sneers and insults.

One careful housewife said, "You can't stay here over night, if you have been with the soldiers you are probably lousy." The unfortunate woman was too nearly exhausted to travel farther that night, and made a bed for herself and children in a stack by the roadside. The night was mild for that season of the year; still they were far from comfortable. They had suffered from frostbitten fingers and toes for some time. On this night hunger was added to their discomforts.

Alfred repeated the little prayer that he had been taught to say before going to bed. But to the mother came the bitter thought, "God has forsaken us."

The next morning as they plodded slowly and painfully along they were overtaken by a farmer who was driving homeward from a neighboring settlement. He spoke kindly and invited them to ride. The invitation was gladly accepted, and the talk of death and suffering was poured into sympathetic ears. He took the wanderers to his home where they rested until the next day, cared for by the good wife.

Late in the month of February (1814) they reached the old homestead, and oh, how warmly the loved daughter was welcomed by her aged parents, who had been very anxious in her behalf. Twelve years before she left that peaceful home a happy bride blessed with health and strength. She returned almost a wreck physically, with mind tortured by fears for her absent loved ones, hardly daring to hope that any of them had escaped death.

For weeks she was very ill, but as the spring advanced and the weather became warm and pleasant a measure of strength and health returned. Alfred and his baby brother became the pets of the household. They were indeed a great comfort to their mother but did not fill the place of the lost ones.

In June glad tidings came. The good Methodist preacher on his way to conference at New York, stopped to inform Orville's grandparents of his safety, and was much surprised to see the mother and brothers of his protégé. "Elder" Glezen Fillmore had become attached to Orville and begged to be allowed to keep him for a time at least.

Months passed, summer fading into autumn and autumn changing to winter, but they brought no news of Miles or his father. The hope that they were still living grew faint, and they were mourned as dead.

A treaty of peace between the United States and Great Britain was signed at Ghent, December 24, 1814. As soon as the news reached America all prisoners of war were set at liberty.

Among those released from Montreal prison was a man of perhaps 45 years. His fine countenance wore a look of sadness and his once glossy brown hair was nearly white. The reader has already guessed his name, Solomon Gillette.

He made a hurried visit to his ruined home at Lewiston, but could find no trace of his family. Then came the impulse to visit his wife's people in Columbia County -- an impulse to which he yielded. The strong man felt the need of sympathy.

It would be impossible to describe the meeting of the husband and wife, who as it seemed to them welcomed each other back from the dead. Their great happiness was mingled with sorrow when they thought of the little boy and the brave youth, who were no more. For Miles was killed by the Indians when Fort Gray was taken.

In a few months the reunited family went back to Lewiston, where they lived for many years. Several children were born to them after the war, but they never ceased to mourn the untimely death of Miles and Jervis.

Lt. Col. E. Cruikshank,
Drummond's 1813 Winter Campaign
Published by Lundy's Lane Historical Society
Second Edition

General Riall had meanwhile crossed the river with 1000 regulars and militia and nearly 500 Western Indians directed by the veterans Matthew Elliott and William Caldwell, who had led the same tribes at the Blue Licks and Sandusky in the Revolution and in many a bloody combat in the present war.[1]

At five o'clock (5am, December 19, 1813) a single cannon shot from Fort Niagara conveyed the welcome tiding that that fortress was in Murray's possession, and the march to Lewiston was begun.

The force stationed there under Major Bennett consisted of a weak regiment of New York State Artillery, numbering 7 officers and 120 men with two guns, and 47 Tuscarora Indians from the neighboring reserve.

As soon as he found his position seriously threatened, Bennett summoned Mallory's battalion of Canadian Volunteers to his aid from Schlosser. His whole force did not then exceed 300, and was rapidly diminished by desertion. He set fire to the public building and attempted to carry off his guns by the Ridge Road. But, being sharply attacked by the light troops and the Indians, these were abandoned and the Americans dispersed in every direction, leaving seventeen dead on the field and a few prisoners.

Unhappily, the Indians broke the solemn pledge exacted from them before crossing the river, and committed numerous outrages. Not only did they ransack and burn every house in sight, including the Tuscarora village, but they seem to have killed and wounded some of the unresisting inhabitants.

The entire number of persons killed has been stated by one writer at forty-six, but this is an evident exaggeration.[2]

---

[1] 8th Regt. and 89th Light Co, 250; 41st, Grenadiers, 100th, 250; Royal Scots, 400; Militia, 100

[2] Chipman P. Turner, Dark Days on the Frontier, mentioned 46 killed.

Twenty-seven women and children were rescued from their hands by the British regulars, one of whom was actually killed by them while protecting the prisoners from their fury. One six and one twelve pounder, a quantity of small arms, nine barrels of powder and 200 barrels of provisions were captured.[1]

---

[1] Cruikshank, Drummond's Winter Campaign, referencing: James' Mil. Occ., vol. II, 19

Louis L. Babcock
The War of 1812 On the Niagara Frontier
Chapter VIII
The Scholar's Bookshelf

The Spoliation of the American Frontier

The destruction of the settlements on the American Frontier had its origin in an outrage perpetrated by the American army while it was stationed at Fort George.

After General Harrison and Colonel Scott left Fort George, General McClure was in an extremely precarious position. On the 17th of November 1813, he wrote the Secretary of War that about four hundred volunteers had joined him, but that the term of service of his troops would expire on the 9th of December, and that if Fort George was to be held the Secretary would see at once the necessity of prompt arrangements being made to reinforce him.

No effective effort was made to aid McClure and he became increasingly apprehensive over his position. On the 4th of October, 1813 General Armstrong, the then secretary of war, had issued the following order to the commanding officer of Fort George:

> War Department, October 4, 1813.
> Sir: Understanding that the defense of the post committed to your charge may render it proper to destroy the Town of Newark, you are hereby directed to apprise its inhabitants of this circumstance and to invite them to remove themselves and their effects to some place of greater safety.

Armstrong expressed himself clearly, and obviously it was the intent of the order that Newark should be destroyed only in the event that a resolute defense of Fort George required it. It was not an authorization to burn the village at will or for any other reason than the one so definitely expressed.

General Vincent, whose excellent work on the Frontier has never received the credit which it deserved, had become ill and obtained leave to return to England. His command was taken over by major General Phineas Riall. Lieutenant-General Sir Gordon Drummond succeeded De-Rottenburg as supreme commander of the forces as well as the head of the civil government of Upper Canada. Drummond was an energetic and resolute soldier and Riall was also a fighter.

When the tension on Montreal was relieved by the failure of Wilkinson's expedition, Prevost directed Drummond to take the offensive whenever the situation warranted it, and that was enough to put Gordon Drummond in motion.

On the 7th of December, Colonel Murray of the British army was ordered to make a reconnaissance as far as Twelve-mile Creek (St. Catharines) with a force of five hundred men and two field guns. Murray, to, was a forceful, aggressive officer.

At Twenty-mile Creek (Jordan) he came in contact with a scouting party of Willcocks' mounted infantry, which he dispersed, and pressing on beyond the point to which he had been ordered, he marched on Fort George.

McClure seems to have been apprised of his approach, for he called a council of war on the question of the advisability of holding the post. The members of the council unanimously favored its abandonment.

Therefore, on the 10th of December, 1813, the inhabitants were informed that the village would be destroyed within two hours. Some removed their furniture; others paid no heed to the warning and soon the snow began to fall and the wind rose to a gale. Late that afternoon a detail was sent out and the work of destruction begun.

Dr. Chapin afterwards asserted that McClure, aided by the renegade Canadian Joseph Willcocks, led the men through the town torch in hand, but Chapin's statements sometimes were highly colored.

On that day, eighty buildings were destroyed and about four hundred women and children were rendered homeless. Many families were denied the support and aid of the normal male population of the village, for the majority of the men were absent from home in the service, or were prisoners in the hands of the Americans. The sick, the old and the infirm all shared in the common misfortune. All the houses were burned save one or two and the loss was appraised later on at about $152,600.

While the village was in flames, McClure wrote the Secretary of War as follows:

> Niagara, December 10, 1813.
> This day found Fort George left to be defended by only sixty effective regular troops under Captains Rogers and Hampton of the 24th Regiment of the United States Infantry and probably forty volunteers. Within the last three days the term of service of the militia has been expiring and they have re-crossed the river almost to a man. Foreseeing the defenseless situation in which the fort was left, I had authorized some of my most active subalterns to raise volunteer companies for two months and offered a bounty in addition to the month's pay.
>
> It is with regret I have to say that this expedient failed of producing the desire effect. A very inconsiderable number were willing to engage for a further term of service on any conditions.
>
> From the most indubitable information I learn that the enemy are advancing in force. This day a scouting party of Colonel Willcocks' volunteers came in contact with the advance at the Twelve Mile Creek, lost four prisoners and one killed; one of the former they gave up to the savages. This movement determined me in calling a council of the principal regular and militia officers left at Fort George this morning.

They all accorded in opinion that the fort was not tenable with the remnant of force left in it. I in consequence gave orders for evacuating the fort and since dusk and with but three boats have brought over all the light artillery and most of the arms, equipage, ammunition, etc., and shall doubtless have time to dispose of the heavy cannon before the enemy makes his appearance.

The village of Newark is not in flames; the few remaining inhabitants in it having been notified of our intention were enabled to remove their property. The houses were generally vacant long before. This step has not been taken without counsel and is in conformity with the views of Your Excellency disclosed to me in a former communication.

The enemy are now completely shut out from any hopes or means of wintering in the vicinity of Fort George.

It is truly mortifying to me that a part of the militia at least could not have been prevailed on to continue in service for a longer term, but the circumstance of their having to live in tents at this inclement season, added to that of the paymaster coming on only prepared to furnish them with one out of thee months pay has had all the bad effects that can be imagined. The best and most subordinate militia that have yet been on the frontier, finding that their wages were not ready for them, became with some meritorious exceptions, a disaffected and ungovernable multitude.

December 11th. I have this moment received a communication from the Governor of this State, covering a requisition on Major General Hall for one thousand men. It is probable that not more than six or seven hundred will rendezvous on this frontier which will in my humble opinion be not more than competence to its proper protection as some will have to be stationed at Black Rock, Schlosser and Lewiston.

I have written to General P. B. Porter desiring him to employ the Indians for the protection of Buffalo until the detachment arrives. Our shipping is in danger. No exertion will be wanting within the pale of our limited means to afford the protection contemplated.

It will be observed that the only reason McClure assigned for his act was to prevent the British army from being housed at Newark during the winter, which admittedly was beyond any instructions that he had received.

After darkness had settled down, Colonel Murray saw the reflection of the burning village written in the sky and swiftly marched to the scene of the conflagration, which he reached about nine o'clock that evening. Fort George had then been evacuated but the fortifications were found to be intact. McClure had taken only some of the lighter guns over the river and the rest were discovered in the ditches of the fort when daylight came. Murray reported that one of the magazines had been blown up but that the smaller ones had been left untouched. Tents for fifteen hundred men were left standing, together with all the barracks. As a matter of fact, the inhabitants of the town had several hours' notice to secure their household property, but viewed in any aspect, the destruction of this fine village was cruel and unjustifiable.

On December 13th, Drummond reached York where he learned that his forces were in possession of Fort George, so he hastened to the Niagara, which he reached on the 16th. On December 14th he wrote the following letter to General McClure:

York, 14th December 1813

Sir: Lieutenant-General Drummond, President and commanding the forces in Upper Canada, having just received a report from the officer in command of the British troops on the Niagara Frontier that the whole of the town of Niagara was destroyed by fire previous to its being evacuated by the American troops, I am directed to call upon you immediately and distinctly to state whether this atrocious act has been committed by the authority of the American Government or is the unauthorized act of any individual. It is essential that not a moment should be lost in returning a specific answer to this communication.

After the destruction of our entire frontier, General Wilkinson by direction of the President disavowed the act of McClure in the following communication to Sir George Prevost:

Plattsburg, January 28th, 1814

Sir: I am commanded by the Executive of the United States to disavow the conduct of Brigadier-General McClue of the militia of the State of New York in burning the town of Newark and in irrefragable testimony that this act was unlicensed to transmit to Your Excellency a copy of the order under color of which that officer perpetrated a deed abhorrent to every American feeling. From this testimonial Your Excellency will perceive that the authority to destroy the village was limited expressly to the defense of Fort George, a measure warranted by the laws of modern war and justified by precedents innumerable.

The outrages which have ensued upon the unwarrantable destruction of Newark have been carried too far and present the aspect rather of vindictive fury than just retaliation, yet they are imputed more to personal feeling than any settled plan of policy deliberately weighed and adopted, and I hope I shall receive from Your Excellency an assurance that this conclusion is not fallacious, for although the wanton conflagrations on the waters of the Chesapeake are fresh in the recollection of every citizen of the United States, no system of retaliation which has for its object the devastation of private property, will ever be resorted to by the American Government but in the last extremity, and this will depend on the conduct of your royal master's troops in this country.

The country unsparingly criticized McClure's conduct. A resident of Manlius was present at the burning of the town and a letter from him dated December 11th, 1813, was published in his home paper. As it probably reflected the view of McClure's own men, it is here set forth:

Last evening General McClure ordered Fort George and Newark to be set on fire which was done. The fort was totally destroyed and the village shared the same fate excepting one or two houses which were spared for the night on the condition that the owners would fire them the next day. The destruction and misery which this dastardly conduct has occasioned is scarcely to be described, women and children being the principal inhabitants have nowhere to place their heads.

McClure after remaining two days at Fort Niagara left for Buffalo. Before his departure he issued orders to Captain Leonard, the commanding officer, which indicated that he believed the British would attack the fort at an early day. He warned Leonard to be extremely vigilant and ready for an attack. His movements from that time on are involved in doubt, but apparently Buffalo gave him a hostile reception. We find him at Williamsville and then in Batavia and Canandaigua engaged in a futile attempt to gather men for the defense of the frontier which he had abandoned.

The following letter by McClure, written on Christmas, the original of which is now before me, discloses the reception he met with at Buffalo when he reached that place. Five days later Buffalo was in flames.

Batavia, 25 December, 1813.
To Col. Erastus Granger.
Dear Sir: I rec'd a letter from Major Mallory wherein he states Buffalo to be still in danger. I should say there is at least twelve hundred men now at that place. I believe the reason that the enemy is concentrating their forces at Erie is that they are apprehensive of your attacking them or why come up there to pass over when they have the command of the river below.

I have requested Major Gen. Hall to take the command of the volunteers & other troops at Buffalo a few days until I organize a detachment of militia. I will send all the troops on as fast as they arrive. The officers commanding the regulars will not return to Buffalo until compelled by a positive order. I should not urge them unless the place is actually in danger.

I would not prevail upon them to stay at Eleven Mile Creek nor was it safe for me or any that accompanied me to stay there or travel the road. The numerous mob that we met all cried out, 'shoot him, damn him; shoot him.'

This mob is countenanced by many of the inhabitants of Buffalo and I must be well convinced that they will treat me in a different way before I can agree to make that my headquarters.

I am under many obligations to you Col. for your stable friendship towards me. I am publishing a hand bill which I will send to you and will be pleased to have you distribute. It is a narrative of facts, which will justify me in the eyes of every impartial man. The detachment of militia will be on at Buffalo in a few days after which I presume the volunteers will return home. I have wrote the Governor that a detachment of one thousand men more would actually be necessary this winter, or regular soldiers.

I am obliged to stop short, with assurances of my highest consideration and esteem and believe me yours sincerely,
                              Geo. McClure.

Tell Captain Hull that now is his time to enlist volunteers. Please do write me occasionally how you come. After I organize the detachment and send them on I shall go home for a few days.

The last letter from McClure in my possession was written to Erastus Granger from Batavia on December 28th. He there states that he proposes visiting his family:

> The gross insults which I have received from
> many at Buffalo will apologize for my absence.
> When I return again with regular troops I will be
> enabled to do myself ample justice.

Some three years afterward, Lieutenant Francis Hall of the British army passed through Bath where McClure lived and he related at an inhabitant of Newark had recovered a judgment against McClure for $1400 in a trial held at Canandaigua, based on McClure ordering the destruction of property the plaintiff owned at Newark. I have not been able to verify this interesting fact for the court records have been dispersed.

Newark had been the capital of Upper Canada and was associated in the mind of every loyal Canadian with the early struggles of the province and the names of Simcoe and Brock. Its wanton destruction under these circumstances and in this season of the year naturally called for stern and immediate measures of retribution; and Drummond instantly put them in train. Naturally his thoughts turned to the capture of the ancient fortress of Fort Niagara only nine hundred yards away, then garrisoned by about three hundred and fifty men under the command of Captain Leonard of the regular army.

The day after his arrival, British Lt. Gen. Drummond issued the following order to Colonel John Murray (written by Lt. Col. Harvey):

> St. David's, December 17, 1813
> Sir: It appearing to Lieutenant-General
> Drummond that the present moment is highly
> favorable for an attack on Fort Niagara, I am
> directed to acquaint you that the Lieutenant-
> General has selected you to command the force
> to be employed on this service, and to add that it

is his wish that the attack should be made this night if possible.The 100th Regiment, the Grenadiers of the Royals, the flank companies 41st Regiment and a party of Royal Artillery are the troops placed at your disposal and you will be pleased to make such a disposal of them for the attack as you may think proper. The remainder of the regular troops, with the whole body of the Indians, will be passed over to support you.

It is hoped that, with the bateaux just arrived from the head of the lake, you may be able to pass over the whole of the attacking troops in two embarkations, and by this means effect a surprise. It is further hoped that a sufficient number of militiamen will come forward as volunteers, not only to man the bateaux for the purpose of bringing them back to this shore, (as soon as the first embarkation shall have been effected), but also for which purpose it should be recommended that every militia volunteer should come provided with a sharp axe.

The troops should carry scaling ladders (at least eighteen or twenty) and should be divided into at least two attacks, one to be made on the lake face and the other on the river. The troops must preserve the profoundest silence and the strictest discipline. They must on no account be suffered to load without the orders of their officers. It should be impressed on the mind of every man that the bayonet is the weapon on which the success of the attack must depend.

J. Harvey, Lt.-Col., D.A.G.

N.B.

100th Regiment (say)	350
Royals	100
41st	100
Royal Artillery	12
	562

The boats to carry the detachment were procured from Burlington Bay and secreted between the fort and Queenston. On the night of December 18th, Murray embarked his force and landed on the American shore near Youngstown early during the following morning. Here the Americans had a picket and half way to the fort was another. The morning was very cold with a strong wind and the ground was covered with snow. The sentries were not at their posts so that the British were able to capture both pickets, numbering forty men, without firing a shot. They were bayonetted to a man, but the watchword was secured before putting them all to death. The British planned to attack in three columns. One attack was directed against the main gate, another was to scale the eastern demi-bastions, and a third the salient angle.

A lieutenant in the 100th Regiment in later years vividly described the approach of the British as follows:

> There lay between them and their destination a small hamlet, called Youngstown, about two miles, or somewhat less, from the fort, to which it served as an outpost, where it was known lay a detachment from the garrison.

> It was necessary to surprise it without alarming the fort.

> A chosen body was therefore sent in advance, while the main body followed at a convenient distance.

When arrived near it, some of the former crept
stealthily up to a window and peeped in. They
saw a party of officers at cards. "What are
trumps?" one of them asked. "Bayonets are
trumps!" answered one of the peepers, breaking
in the window and entering with his
companions, while the remainder of the
detachment rapidly surrounded the house,
rushed into it and bayoneted the whole of its
inmates, that none might escape to alarm the
fort. Not a shot was fired on either side, the
American sentries having retired from their
posts into a building to shelter themselves from
the cold, there was not time for resistance.

The assailants performed their work of human
destruction in grim silence – a lamentable but
necessary act.

Resuming their march, they drew near the fort –
not a word is spoken – the muskets are carried
squarely, that the bayonets may not clash – the
ice crackles audibly under their tread, but the
sound is borne to their rear on the continuous
gusts of a northeast wind – when lo! The
charger of Colonel Hamilton (who, having lost a
leg in Holland, could not march, and would not
stay behind) neighs loudly and is answered by a
horse in a stable not far from the fort. What a
moment! The force instantly halts, expecting to
hear the alarm suddenly given, the sound of
drums and bugles and of the garrison rushing to
their posts. But all remains quiet, the sentries,
crouching in their boxes, take the neigh of the
charger for that of some horse strayed from a
farmhouse or the neighboring hamlet. They feel
no inclination for leaving their shelters to

explore, shiveringly, the thick darkness of a
moonless winter night.

It can be nothing. The approaching force,
drawing freer breath, put itself in motion,
shuffles hastily and silently forward and the
crisis is near.

As the British were moving into position the main gate of
the fort was opened to change the guard on the water front so they
were able to gain the barrack square without opposition. They met
with some resistance elsewhere but in a few moments the work
was complete and at 5am on December 19, the fort was again in
the hands of the British were it remained till the close of the war.
Leonard was visiting his family four miles away at the time.

The British did not fire a shot.

The American loss by the bayonet was sixty-five killed,
fourteen were wounded and three hundred and forty-four were
taken prisoners, making an aggregate of four hundred and twenty-
three. The British loss was six killed and five wounded. The
capture of this important post was a severe blow to the Americans
for it was an entrepot for the frontier.

Some idea of its importance may be gained from the
following report on its contents, made by Drummond to Prevost a
few days after the assault.

Arms, about four thousand stand, with capital
accoutrements, principally new, to the same
amount. An immense quantity of musket
ammunition. Seven thousand and one hundred
and fifty pairs of shoes. The clothing of the
Kings and 49th Regiments. An immense
quantity of American clothing of every
description, and also necessaries in equal
abundance. Many thousand pairs of blankets
and great-coats. Camp equipage, medical
stores, wine, tea, forges with armourer's tools,

salt, spirits, beef, flour, paper, etc. The value of
the captured property, including the guns and
their stores, it is supposed, cannot amount to
less than one hundred and fifty-thousand to two
hundred thousand pounds. Independent of the
stores found in the fort several boat loads of
valuable articles were taken at the Four Mile
Creek, where they had been sent the day before
the assault.

The fort was well garrisoned and well found in everything
essential to its defense, and its commander knew that an attack was
imminent. Its loss was the result either of gross negligence or
treason, and its retention by the British during the remainder of the
war was a source of embarrassment to our commissioners during
the negotiation of the Treaty of Ghent. The small proportion of
wounded to the killed tells the story of the ruthlessness of the
British attack. Drummond's report follows:

Fort Niagara, 20th Dec., 1813.
Sir: Conceiving the possession of Fort Niagara
to be of the highest importance, in every point
of view, to the tranquility and serenity of this
frontier, immediately on my arrival at St.
David's, I determined upon its reduction, if
possible without too great a sacrifice. There
being, however, but two bateaux on this side the
water, I did not think proper to make the attempt
until a sufficient number should be brought from
Burlington, at this season of the year a most
difficult undertaking.

But, by the indefatigable exertions of Captain
Eliot, Deputy Assistant Quartermaster General,
every difficulty, particularly in the carriage of
the bateaux by land for several miles,
notwithstanding the inclemency of the weather,

(the ground being covered with snow, and the frost severe), was overcome; they were again launched, and the troops, consisting of a small detachment of the Royal Artillery, the grenadier company of the Royal Scots, the flank companies of the 41st and the 100th Regiment, amounting in the whole to about five hundred and fifty, which I had placed under the immediate orders of Colonel Murray, Inspection Field Officer, were embarked.

The enclosed report of that most zealous and judicious officer will point out to you the detail of their further proceedings.

At 5 o'clock a.m. the fort was attacked by assault, at the point of the bayonet, two picquets, posted at the distance of a mile and of a mile and a half from the works, having previously been destroyed to a man by the same weapon, and in half an hour afterwards this important place was completely in our possession.

By this gallant achievement twenty-seven pieces of ordnance (mounted on the several defenses), three thousand stands of arms, a number of rifles, a quantity of ammunition, blankets, clothing several thousand pairs of shoes, etc., have fallen into our hands, besides fourteen officers and 330 other prisoners, and eight respectable inhabitants of this part of the country, who had been dragged from the peaceful enjoyment of their property to a most unwarrantable confinement were released, together with some Indian warriors of the Cocknawaga and Six Nation tribes. The

enemy's loss amount to sixty-five in killed and
to but twelve in wounded, which clearly proves
how irresistible a weapon the bayonet is in the
hands of British soldiers.

While the force of Colonel Murray was marching on Fort
Niagara, General Riall with about one thousand regulars and a
large force of western Indians also crossed the river.

When Murray signaled that the fort had fallen, Riall
advanced on Lewiston where a small force of militia and a few
Indians were stationed. The Americans after destroying a quantity
of public property attempted to retreat with some of the artillery,
but they were soon dispersed by the Indians with a loss of
seventeen killed and an unknown number wounded.

It appears from Riall's report that his troops did not come
in contact with the Americans who seemed to have been driven off
by the Indians. General Drummond was apprehensive over the
employment of Indians for such duty and before the expeditions
were sent over he exacted promises from the chiefs that they would
refrain from their usual savage practices.

In the attack on Lewiston, they broke away from all
restraint and used the tomahawk and scalping knife upon the dead,
the wounded and the unhurt, irrespective of sex or age.
Drummond says in his report to Prevost:

> I reported to your Excellency that the Indians
> who advanced with Major General Riall's force
> on the morning of the 19th had committed great
> excesses in consequence of intoxication and had
> burnt the greatest part of the houses at or near
> Lewiston. I have now the honor to state that on
> withdrawing the troops from Lewiston
> yesterday (Dec. 22) I thought it advisable, the
> inhabitants having in general quitted their
> houses, to direct the remainder of them to be set
> on fire in order to deprive the enemy of cover
> for troops that might be sent for the purpose of

destroying the opposite town of Queenston.

Such were the curt and official words of General Drummond used in describing the atrocities of these western Indians. An unknown American officer writing to the Albany Argus newspaper on December 26, 1813, paints the scene at Lewiston in more graphic language:

> The Indians then began their hellish work by burning the buildings and plundering, killing and scalping the inhabitants. On the river and from six to eight miles on the Ridge Road they have not left a house from the fort to Schlosser except one owned by Mr. Fairbanks a Federalist of the Boston stamp. On Friday I proceeded with thirty mounted volunteers to Lewiston. The sight we here witnessed was shocking beyond description.
>
> Our neighbors were seen lying dead in the field and roads, some horribly cut and mangled with tomahawks, other eaten by the hogs which were probably left for that purpose, as they were almost the only animals found alive.
>
> It is not yet ascertained how many were killed as most of the bodies were thrown into the burning houses and consumed.

We have another graphic description of the destruction of the settlement from the pen of Jonas Harrison, the collectors of customs for the District of Niagara, who wrote his official chief from Batavia on December 24, 1813:

> Sir: On Sunday morning the 19th inst. The British landed unobserved about 900 Indians and 600 or 700 Regulars at the Five Mile

Meadow about half way between Lewiston and
Fort Niagara... They showed themselves at
Lewiston about sunrise and strange to tell we
had not more than three to five minutes notice of
their being on our side before their Indians were
at my house. They, as far as we can learn (for it
is said they are still in possession of the country)
commenced an indiscriminate slaughter of men,
women and children together with burning
every house, barn, outhouse and hovel that
could take fire.

The citizens about Lewiston and its vicinity
below the slope or highland that form the Falls
of Niagara, escaped by the Ridge Road towards
Genesee Falls, all going the one road on foot,
old and young, men, women, and children flying
from their beds, some not more than half
dressed, without shoes or stockings, together
with men on horseback, wagons, carts, sleighs
and sleds overturning and crushing each other,
stimulated by the horrid yells of the 900 savages
on the pursuit, which lasted eight miles, formed
a scene awful and terrific in the extreme.

The small military force we had were the first to
fly... We have lost our all and the scene is over.

This description is overdrawn but judging from the British
reports it must have been based on facts.

In those days sober Indians were bad enough; drunken
savages must have been fiendish in their ferocity.

Elias Johnson
Legends, Traditions and Laws of the Iroquois of Six Nations and the History of the Tuscarora, 1881

The Tuscaroras again evinced their friendship for the United States in the war of 1812, when they were asked to guard the Niagara River at Lewiston and down the river, against the British crossing it.

Here again we hear of the Tuscarora sachem, Solomon Longboard, with about thirty-five Tuscarora volunteers, stationed at Lewiston on guard. I have recorded some of the names of these volunteers, which I was able to obtain from some of the old people that were yet living in the year 1878, which are as follows, to-wit: The two sons of Solomon Longboard, Jacob Taylor, Joseph Cusick, John Cusick, David Cusick, John Black Nose and his brother, Samuel Thompson, John Obediah, Aaron Pempleton, James Pempleton, John Mt. Pleasant, Harry Patterson, John Green, Issac Allen, Capt. Williams, Gau-ya-re-na-twa, Wm. Printup better known as little Billy, Black Chief, John Printup, Issac Green, Surgin Green, George Printup. There were but few of these that drew pension, as it was alleged that they were not enrolled upon the army roll.

On the night of December 19th, 1813[1], the British army and the British Indians crossed the Niagara River near Calvin Hotchkis' place, about two miles below Lewiston. They noticed at first there were lights going across the river during the night, and at the dawn of day were dispatched, Jacob Taylor (better known as Colonel Jacobs), and another Indian to accompany him – both being Tuscaroras. On their return they reported that the British Indians had crossed the river in great numbers. The news was circulated in the village of Lewiston and the neighboring country, that they might evacuate their places and go east, which they did, taking the Ridge Road. The Tuscarora volunteers took the rear of

---

[1] The crossing took place the evening before, on December 18, 1813. The attack was early in the morning on December 19.

the train as they moved eastward, commanded by their Sachem, Solomon Longboard.

The British Indians went on the pursuit. After they had gone about two miles from the village of Lewiston, where the Tuscarora Indians branched off on a road leading to their reservation, known as the Indian hill, or Mountain Road. As they had advanced part way up the mountain they observed a Canada Indian on horseback, who headed off some of the train, and among the rest was also Bates Cooke, of Lewiston. One of his legs had, a little previous to that time, been amputated, and the main Canada force were about half a mile in the rear on pursuit. The commander of the Tuscarora force ordered that the Indian heading off the train be shot, which was done by John Obediah. The Indian tumbles off the horse and fell to the ground, and then got up and ran down the little hill into the wood, where it is said he died from the wound he received.

When the report of the gun was heard by the Canadian force and they saw the effect it had on their comrade, they halted. Their commander, Mr. Longboard, of the Tuscaroras which numbered at that time twenty-six, from them selected three men and instructed them to get upon and to go along the top of the mountain and to blow a horn occasionally, which they had in their possession, and to keep nearly opposite the Canada Indians.

The object was to serve as a scarecrow, to make them believe that there was a force also on the mountain in the act of flanking them.

But the remaining force of Mr. Longboard rushed down the mountain with their war whoops as if legion were coming down, and pursued the Canada Indians, while the train of white people had gone on in their flight. The Canada Indians retreated about one mile and a half, near to where the main force were.

Then one of their men halted and aimed his gun at one of our men, John Obediah, and the latter also aimed to his opponent, while Samuel Thompson got behind a large elm tree. In the meantime, John Obediah spoke to the stranger in all the different six languages of the Iroquois, but did not get an answer. These were the only two men in pursuit at this time, as the rest of them had halted some ways back.

Finally the British Indian retreated backwards, keeping aim as he went, and all at once gave a spring and ran off. The three men that were on the mountain kept occasionally blowing the horn as they went, as the road is parallel with the mountain.

By this time the train of white people had gone quite a good ways in their flight: it is evident that the timely intervention of the Tuscarora Indians, saved great slaughter of men, women and children among the white people.

The Tuscaroras then went back and kept in the rear of the white people in their flight. The British Indians perceiving that it was the Tuscarora Indians that killed one of their number and repulsed them, made their way to the reservation, (the nation had already deserted their homes), and began to burn their houses indiscriminately, and also a meeting-house which was built by them, except eight dollars, a convenient chapel where the early Christian Tuscaroras such as Sacaresa and Solomon Longboard, both sachems, with many others, delighted to worship the Almighty in the simplicity of their faith.

And after they had finished their destruction they went down in pursuit of the fleeing train of white people on the ridge road: by this time the Tuscaroras had stationed themselves at a log house, eight or ten miles from Lewiston, near Nathan Peterson's, which was used as an armory; when the Tuscaroras first came, there were a few white men there breaking open the powder kegs in this log house, making it ready to set on fire but the chief, Mr. Longboard, remonstrated in having it burned, and was interpreted to them by Colonel Jacobs, so they consented not to destroy the powder.

When the British Indians came in sight, Mr. Longboard instructed his men to keep moving back and forth from the log house or armory, to a thicket in the rear of the house, for the purpose of making the enemy believe that there was a large force stationed there; the enemy halted and finally went back, and thus the armory was saved.

The maneuver of the Tuscarora Indians in these two cases above, was done with but very little sacrifice on their part, but the beneficence was great; but then, who cares anything about that, it was nothing but an Indian affair anyhow; this will probably be the thought of those who peruse my little pages.

Joshua Cooke (son of Bates Cooke)
Reminiscences of Lewiston
Souvenir History of Niagara County, New York
Commemorative of the 25th Anniversary of The Pioneer
Association of Niagara County, 1902

Escape from the Indians

Then came, in 1813, the catastrophe following McClure's barbarous act of burning Newark on his evacuation. In vengeance, the fort was taken, and British and Indians, spread along the river, burning and murdering all in their way. One after another, nearly a dozen were shot down. A. Millar and S. Gillette were taken prisoners to Montreal, not returning till the next year. The case of Dr. Alvord was pitiful. He was a cripple, and, attempting to escape on horseback, was shot down and tomahawked. When he was found his poor fingers were slit down to the wrists with the hatchets, as he had vainly held them up to parry the blows or to ask for mercy. Dr. Willard Smith escaped on foot, and was, incidentally, the means of the escape of all the male members of my grandfather's family. It will not be deemed too much that I should give an account of this; it has been often printed, and I will give it as it is known in our family

My uncle, Lothrop Cooke, had lost his leg in hauling Van Rensselaer's boat through the cold water to a point where they could make Hennepin's Rock in the fight. He was in the last stage of weakness, and the least motion was feared as endangering his life. News came to the home, east of the village about a mile, of the taking of the Fort and the coming of the Indians. Sending the women of the family ahead with the horses, my grandfather yoked his oxen to a sled; covered it with straw and blankets, and my father carried the helpless one out in his arms.

He survived the moving, and the little band of father and three sons started for the road, going east. My father had a musket; there were no other arms.

Dr. Smith came along on foot, and said, "Bates, is your gun loaded?"

"No, I have no cartridges."

"Well, I have two, load your gun with one and I will load mine with the other." And he passed on.

They had arrived at the hollow, where the road to the Reservation turns off, up the mountain, where five British Indians came up rapidly on horseback. The chief had a sword in place of a hatchet, and riding up behind the sleigh, he made a pass at my uncle, but his blow fell short.

My uncle has told me of his feeling at the moment. He was so weak that he could not turn his head to avoid the sword, and thought his end had come. A brass kettle, hanging on the hind sled stake rattled just then; the horses started back, and the savage missed his blow.

He rode up again, when my father raised his gun and fired. My uncle said that he was looking up directly in the Indian's face, when the bullet struck him in the throat, a gush of flood followed, he wheeled and fell, rose up and ran a few rods and fell dead.

The other Indians had fired a random volley to break my father's aim, at which a little band of friendly Tuscaroras in the mountain, but hidden by trees, fired a random volley, and gave the war whoop. They were led by the noted little Col. Jacobs.

The attacking party, alarmed, spurred their horses into the woods for Fort Niagara.

The sleigh had gone about a mile when Mr. Sparrow Sage overtook it and said, "Bates, the Indian's horse has run into my yard; you had better go back for him; it will help you all away."

He did so.

His little office and his few books had been burned on his return; he sold the horse for sixty dollars, and it was his beginning in life again. One of his first suits in court was in defense of title to the horse. The horse had been captured from soldiers by the Indian and had the "United States" brand upon him. A government commissary saw the brand and claimed him. The plea was made that the horse had been captured by the enemy and belonged to any person who should retake him from the enemy. It was declared good law, and the purchaser kept the horse.

The larger things of life lie in the smaller. Dr. Smith's single cartridge and Jacob's war whoop held in them the life of our family, and the sixty dollars was the beginning of a practice which ended in Congress and the Comptrollership at Albany. But the latter did what the Indian hatchet could not do; it killed him!

After the war most of the settlers came back in one or two years. Many others followed; the town, the county, were organized, and as it was for long the county town, perhaps more than the average proportion of marked men settled it.

Edited by William Pool
History of Lewiston, New York
Landmarks of Niagara County, NY, Chapter XVII, 1897

When the invasion was made no place on the frontier suffered more than Lewiston. The attack was a surprise. The Indians, preceded by the British a few minutes and under the license given them by Riall, their commander, they began the indiscriminate shooting of the people.

The little force under Major Bennett, that was stationed at the settlement, were soon compelled to retreat after losing a number of men. A few days earlier a small force of Americans and friendly Indians had been gathered for the defense of the frontier between Lewiston and Five mile Meadow; but they were likewise surprised in an unorganized condition and forced to flee. It was in this party that the elder Gillette was engaged, as before related. Soon the only thought on the part of the inhabitants was how to reach a place of safety. An "Old Pioneer" wrote the Lockport Journal a few years ago, as follows:

> At one time when the red-coats were seen landing at Lewiston, every owner of a horse hitched up to his sleigh and piled in their goods and escaped to the mountain. But one woman was left alone in her cabin. As two "reds" came to the house they seized her infant child which happened to be outside and threatened to kill it if she refused to let them in. But she persisted. They dashed the child's brains out against the corner of the house, and then mounting the roof and began descending the chimney. With quick presence of mind she emptied her straw bed into the fire which smothered them so that she easily finished them with her axe. After washing the soot off their faces she recognized two of her neighbors who were Tories.

The killed at Lewiston numbered about twelve, among whom was Dr. Alvord. the pioneer physician, Thomas Marsh, Jervis Gillette, who was only seven years old and who was shot while trying to escape with his mother, and two others named Tiffany and Finch. All but one were scalped and that one was beheaded. Dr. Alvord had just mounted his horse before his dwelling to ride away, but was shot before going far. The escape of Lothrop Cooke and his brother, Bates Cooke, has been narrated.

Reuben Lewis lived at the foot of the mountain on the outskirts of the present village, and having agreed with a neighbor that he would never be taken alive, he fought after he was wounded until the enemy came up and killed him.

The Tuscarora village shared the fate of Lewiston. We quote from Turner as follows:

> The Ridge Road presented one of the harshest features of the invasion. The inhabitants on the frontier, en masse, were retreating eastward, men, women and children, the Tuscarora Indians having a prominent place in the fight. The residents upon the Ridge who had not got the start of the main body, fell in with it as it approached them.

There was a small arsenal at the first four corners west of Howells Creek, a log building containing a number of barrels of powder, several hundred stand of arms and a quantity of fixed ammunition. Making a stop there, the more timid were for firing the magazine and continuing the retreat. The braver counsels prevailed to a small extent. They made sufficient demonstrations to turn hack a few Indian scouts who had followed up the retreat to plunder such as fell in the rear.

The mass made no halt at the arsenal, but pushed on in an unbroken column, until they arrived at Forsythe's, where they divided, a part taking the Lewiston Road and seeking asylums in

Genesee County and over the river, and a part along the Ridge Road and off from it in the new settlements of what are now Orleans and Monroe counties, and Wayne and the north part of Ontario counties.

All kinds of vehicles were put in requisition. It was a motley throng, dying from the torch and the tomahawk of an invading foe, with hardly a show of military organization to cover their retreat.

The enemy pressed on up the river, destroying everything of value on the way. Isaac Colt was wounded at his tavern on the main road toward Niagara Falls. Major Mallory, who seems to have been in command at Fort Schiosser, made a little resistance, but in vain, and the settlement at the falls suffered the fate of Youngstown and Lewiston.

Late in the month (December) a strong force of British went from Fort Niagara east to Wilson and as far as Van Horn's mill in Newfane, destroyed the mill and most of the buildings on their way.

During the following summer, the British being in possession of Fort Niagara, small marauding parties, mostly Indians, paid unwelcome visits to the settlers who had ventured back to their homes.

An Indian who was passing through the woods came out on the Ridge Road at the house of Sparrow S. Sage. Mr. Sage was absent and the house was occupied by his wife and another woman. The Indian took them prisoners and started towards the fort. Before they had proceeded far the companion of Mrs. Sage escaped, found Mr. Sage and told him of the outrage.

He pursued and caught the Indian, wounded him severely and rescued his wife.

Chipman P. Turner
Dark Days on the Frontier of Western New York
Bigelow Bros., 1879

The nineteenth of December, 1813, was a gloomy period; not only for such as were more nearly connected, but for the inhabitants throughout Western New York.

While patriotism had caused the abandonment of homes and all that was dear, to fill the ranks of weak protection, unsuspected treason gained a victory that no other power of the enemy could gain.

During the night of the eighteenth, under the shade of darkness that covered the shame of the perpetrators, the British crossed the Niagara river, at what was then called Pegey's Landing, about one mile below the five-mile meadows; numbering in all, armed soldiers, real and disguised Indians, as estimated, five hundred.

The force of the enemy separated, at this point, into two parties, the one detailed for the Fort constituting the main armed portion, the one for plunder and burning, unarmed, except with torch and hatchet, and a few guns.

The traitor, Nathaniel Leonard, who had been entrusted with the command of the Fort, absented himself, ordering the gates not to be closed, leaving for the enemy an unobstructed entrance. The treachery of Leonard, although not suspected at the time, was a cautiously-devised perfidy, as indicated by using the same password for three nights in succession, adopting his own name as the countersign, enabling an unmolested march into the fort, which Leonard had surreptitiously left neglected for quiet repose on his farm, about two miles distant -- if there could be quietness amid the torturing vision of agonizing, imaginary devils, haunting the bed-chamber occupied by a conscious traitor.

The only resistance was from about one hundred of General Harrison's men, that had been made prisoners after Hull's surrender of Detroit, on the western frontier; having been exchanged and placed in the Fort for hospital treatment. Knowing them to be from the victorious forces of Harrison, antipathy raged to subdue humanity, and most of them are reported to have been massacred.

Col. Murray, with his command, were now the undisputed tenants, without the danger of a forced siege.

There was but little to obstruct the desperation of the party that before day-light had taken the direction of Lewiston without order or discipline, except with the purposes of vagrant desperadoes. Between the landing and Lewiston, the work of destruction was performed during the night.

The next morning there was no one to be found, between the localities, to relate what had happened. All the buildings had been destroyed and the few occupants killed, except the wife and children of a German, that were never seen afterwards -- the father was found dead in the road.

Reaching Lewiston at sunrise, a sudden surprise not only set the inhabitants in commotion, but also caused the precipitate retreat without attempting resistance, of a company of militia, who neither showed a soldier's front, nor stood up to the duty of an armed citizen.

While an indiscriminate slaughter of the confused and fleeing, was enacted by such as had fire-arms, plundering the slain and burning the buildings was the vigorously-performed part of the real and disguised Indians. The most savage cruelty was fiendishly enacted upon such as were unable to escape. The sequel was but another scene of distress and affliction, transpiring in the bloody tragedy.

If any were in or near by hoped-for security, where they could look in dismay upon their consuming homes, the mutilated dead and dying, among whom were the last of neighbors and nearest kindred, the curtain, that had been raised at the dawn of day, dropped before them, to forever cover from sight all that had been held most sacred.

Forty-six were found dead. Of the citizens, whose names have been kept in memory, the following have been furnished: Doctor Alvord, a pioneer physician in Lewiston, Miles Gillette, William Gardener, scalped and head taken off, two brothers by the name of Jones, Helen Mead, Thomas Marsh, Tiffany and Finch; a boy, Gillette, was taken prisoner, and afterwards found dead.

But after a few hours, spent in the worst display of wanton inhumanity, the harsh features of war and sudden invasion were to be visited upon the unprotected inhabitants on the Ridge and the road leading up the mountain to Niagara Falls.

For the purpose in view, the party was again divided. Not anything was to be left in their malicious track; destruction was the fate of everything before them. No check was experienced by the party taking the Ridge Road direction, for nearly two miles; when bravery, the want of which had proved the cowardice of Maj. Bennett and his band of frightened militia, brought a company of armed Tuscaroras to the rescue, led by the war-chief orator Longboard, Col. Johnson, Ovid and Littlegreen. They had heard the alarm and seen the light of the torch, but not the enemy.

Concealed in a favorable thicket, the Tuscaroras awaited the approach of the enemy, and fired a single volley, which sufficiently surprised to cause a retreat and delay, as an advance alarm, that furnished the inhabitants a few lucky minutes to escape from the blow of the tomahawk and thirst of the fatal knife.

At this point was encountered the first resistance, meeting the repulse of death in the ranks of the scouting party; five of which had preceded the main body on horseback; overtaking and ox-team, that was conveying from the scene of death at Lewiston, the invalid, Lothrop Cooke, who a few days before had suffered the amputation of a leg. His brother, Bates Cooke, driving the team, discovering the near approach and murderous design, as the leader advanced in the feathered garb of a war chief, commanded a halt.

The intrepid teamster, in characteristic manner of coolness, that in after years controlled him in private and public life, seized a gun that was upon the sled, and with deliberate aim short the Indian through the neck; who, falling from his horse, died in a few minutes. The fire of the four remaining comrades proving ineffectual to prevent the escape of the brother benefactor with his charge, the terrifying Tuscaroras turned them back among the greater numbers.

The sound of Cooke's gun first brought the Tuscaroras to the ambush, in which they placed themselves in benefactory attitude, that stopped further destruction of life. A few still live, to relate the terrors of that day, of those who experienced the noble act of the Tuscarora braves; and their descendants will keep alive the memory of the deed, which is not the only example of their valor and faithful protection in times of most imminent need.

The repulse was only temporary. Renewing the eager and infernal pursuit, none but vacated houses were found; the death-blow had been stayed by the sudden exit of the inmates, upon whom was intended and early call.

Breakfast tables were found provided with unconsumed warm meals, irregularly-arranged benches and chairs; and indication of the haste in departing. Open doors, though not bidding a kind reception, gave access to possessions abandoned without time to express reluctance. There was but a few minutes' timely notice, to ensure the safety of the eastward retreat of the women and children, accompanied by men; such only as could be spared from the gathering forces, to drive back the hostile intruders.

The rallying point was fixed at the two temporary arsenals, consisting of two log dwellings, that stood on the east and west corners, now owned by Amos B. Gallop (the original foundation is still visible) and Peter Oliphant, on the south ridge, half a mile west of Howell's creek, near where the settlement in the county was first commenced by Philip Beach, in 1801. One of the buildings was used for a deposit of powder, the other for arms.

At the cited locality, Benjamin Barton, Silas Hopkins, Joshua Fairbanks and other citizens, caused a rally of the inhabitants in the vicinity, who were joined by a few of the straggling militia and such as could entrust their fleeing families to others, while they took part in their protection by checking the onward progress of their pursuers.

Arms were placed in the hands of such as it was thought could use them, as they were passing along in the train of the fleeing. As fast as any arrived that could be made serviceable, they were armed, and placed in line, without systematic organization, other than a united determination that proved effectual.

Courage and energy was the voluntary countersign. Thus arrayed, heart and soul inspired, to inflict retributive justice upon the worst of wrongdoers, who had butchered their friends and neighbors, reduced their only homes to ashes, sent them floating at random, destitute wanderers, to seek protection, most of them among strangers, it was felt and known that delay would only prolong the havoc; what was to be done must be done with firm resolve and quickly.

The body of citizens commensurate with the thin population that then existed, were soon on the march to meet and contest face to face, the prerogative of power for further mischief.

Two miles and a half west of the arsenal rendezvous, near the line dividing the towns of Cambria and Lewiston, the vagrant intruders were encountered; the rebut of a single fire, terminated their further advance, scattering them in disorderly retreat, over the ground they had laid waste and strewn with the lifeless remains of their murdered victims, to the protection of Fort Niagara.

On the way to the final terminus of the scouters' mission, two were added to the number of the Lewiston massacred.

Major John Beach, one of the earliest prominent settlers, in attempting the escape of his family, had succeeded with the aid of his hired man, Tiffany, in reaching the place where the Tuscaroras had gathered, before any assault was made upon them, attempting an only hope of escape, concealment in the woods. Tiffany, in consequence of being lame, could endure the fatigue no longer, and exclaiming, "I must stop, if the Indians kill me," was left dead.

The Tuscaroras, witnessing the condition of Beach (detained to aid the less able man), requiting his oft expressed friendship and ready counsel, sprang to his aid, taking him bodily up the mountain, beyond the reach of immediate harm. The family, uninjured, proceeded in the flight.

The practical military qualifications of Major Beach, who had frequently been instructed to drill squads for actual service, probably gave him a position which enabled him to direct in the quick arrangements at the arsenal. The indications of a solitary grave are still pointed out, near where the last repulse took place. It was that of a teamster, Mead, who was conveying household furniture from Lewiston on the morning of the invasions. A single Indian overtook and shot him.

Having followed the branch of the merciless mob that took the route of the Ridge Road, it remains to notice the acts of their associates in villainy who divided off at Lewiston, to make an attack on the few inhabitants upon the mountains. Here the designs were as wicked, the opportunity not as great. There were but a few families they could disturb before reaching the Falls, and there but a commenced settlement.

The statement of a venerable woman, widow of the late Colonel Dickerson, blessed with a retentive memory at the advanced age of eighty-three, is inserted as authentic, she having been a witness:

> My father, Isaac Colt, on the morning of the nineteenth of December, 1813, I think about sunrise, was alarmed at the noise he heard below the mountain; and discovering the smoke rising from the burning buildings, joined by Samuel Hopkins, went on horseback to the brow of the precipice, only to witness the most heartrending scene, in the valley below, that but a few minutes time allowing them to ponder.

> Suddenly surprised by the appearance of several Indians coming from their concealment in the bushes, a quick exit was the dictate of prudence. They urged their horses to the best of speed, for a safe escape. Col. Hopkins riding out of reach was not harmed. When my father reached the house, we found five ball holes in his garments. A ball had made quite a deep skin wound on

his hip, the blood from which had partly
filled his shoe.

The attention of my father and Hopkins was
at once directed towards providing for the
escape of their own and other families, to be
perfected before the destroyers had time to
arrive. It was done so hurriedly that but
little regard was had for what clothing was
worn or hastily tied up in a bundle -- without
even providing a school children's dinner,
for a journey that had no certain end. I got
on board the lumber wagon of a stranger,
that was standing before our door, taking the
younger children in charge. Hertzel and
Alexander D. descended the mountain by
way of the Indian village, expecting to stop
at Solomon Hersey's tavern at
Dickersonville, but found it deserted, as
were all the other houses on Ridge Road.
There was no other way left for me but to
accept the offer of the stranger to be our
benefactor. He carried us during the day and
late in the evening, forty miles east on the
ridge, where we were left to seek an
opportunity to get through to Bristol,
Ontario County, the point I had fixed my
mind upon. I was then 18 years old, and
made my adopted home a residence for
many years afterwards. My father's, with
all the neighbors' buildings were burnt.
John March and one by the name of Frink
were killed.

The narrative thus far is but the "beginning of the end." A
young population had just begun to construct homes, where
civilized effort had not before been made. Eleven years from the

very first settlement did not make the most industrious to see more than a beginning. The majority were inter-medial beginners, many of them of not more than a year or two's standing. The title of citizenship was restricted by the prevalence of woodmen and foresters. Whatever then they had already endured, no forecast enabled them to judge of the crisis forced upon them.

A retreat was made of what there was of a whole community, mingled with the Tuscarora Indian families -- thronging the only way of land escape, the but partially established Ridge Road, to gain an eastern retreat, away from the frontier. The task to relate in language suitable to transmit more than a vague realization, is a difficult one.

Consternation prevailed, beyond the control of the most cautious and deliberate. Men, women and children were to be seen, in half clothed or almost naked condition, tramping in the snow, barefooted, creeping on their hands and knees, for concealment; turning from partly devoured meals, and hastily gathering the little that could be obtained, as a reserve against the famishing hunger of themselves and children. At one time, five infant children, from their mothers' breasts, were found upon the ox sled of John Robinson, placed there by mothers anxious to save their offspring, who adopted this as the only resort for their protection, to save them from the slaughter or a life among savages. The mothers were following in cold dripping garments, to claim their own when the sled was overtaken. The wearied oxen enabled the mothers a part of the time to keep within hailing and approaching distance, to hurriedly embrace them in anxious hope of ultimate, undisturbed reunion.

Families remaining at their but recently provided homes, under the existing state of threatening disaster, had but little hope of prolonged life, or the preservation of the small property they owned; which, yielding a comfortable maintenance, prudence, or, it may be more properly said, necessity, required them to abandon to escape the tomahawk and scalping knife. This was not done until Fort Niagara's defense became a stronghold of the enemy. Fleeing, the tramp of the merciless was on their track. They had only to listen, the savage war-whoop was in hailing distance -- to look back to see the busily applied torch, lighting the paths of precipitate; unprepared for flight.

The late Andrew Robinson, who was a boy teamster, ten years old at this time, previous to his death gave the writer, with many other particulars, the following:

> When we arrived at Wright's Corners, fifteen miles from where we started, it was a little after dark. We could locate the place of our destroyed tenements, as we saw the consuming flames and smoke mingle with the morning clouds. Hungry, we longed for the least remains of the meals we had left behind; my mother, brothers and sisters, too, fatigued beyond endurance for any further progress in our flight that night, could only wish for the poorest bed left behind, to occupy as a couch in the woods. It was a sleepless night, and one of deep despair.
>
> The shade of the dark cloud that hung over our heads cast no greater gloom than the forebodings of the future. The most encouraging hope that could be entertained, was, that should a return even transpire, it would be to ponder over ashen remains, where there was nothing left to satisfy hunger or check the beseeching importunities of crying children.
>
> Where there were former neighbors, peaceably enjoying each other's friendly associations and united efforts, a dismal waste only would be seen; many that were there, were there no more forever.

There were only a portion of the flowing tide that was falling back, seeking asylums in former localities, leaving barren of population the region they had spent their energies to improve. It proved to be a "set back" that took many years to overcome.

During the balance of the winter a few remained; among them Silas Hopkin, Isaac Colt and others, returned to act as patrolling watchmen, over what little might be picked up and saved. It was a lean gathering. Not much could be done to replenish war arrangements for re-inhabiting. The only alternative was to wait for the uncertain events of war, that still remained in threatening aspect.

The next thing an attempt was made for reinstatement, and as far as could be done, to erect temporary dwellings and clear small patches of land.

The following are remembered as returning during the spring (1814) and next season with their families:

John Beach, living in Lewiston, who owned the first farm west
His brothers, Philip and Jesse Beach
John Lattey
Isaac Cook
Sparrow Sage
John Robinson
Rufus Spaulding
Henry Totten
Conrad Bartemus
Ray Marsh
William Enos
Coushin Smith
Aaron Childs
Eli Harris
Achis Pool
Stephen Warren

William Molyneux (at the Corners)[1]

John Gould and William Howell and family did not leave.

For about a year, such as did return could, but feel that they were laboring under an impending protest, that might at any time place them in jeopardy. They endured the continual annoyance of apprehension, until the forepart of the year following, suffering nothing more than thievish plunder. Dismal as the harassing could have been, it was not dispelled for a future clear sky, that could be relied upon for peace and quietness.

---

[1] Molyneaux Corners is known to be at Rt. 104 (Ridge Road) and Plank Road in the Town of Cambria, about 11 miles east of the Village of Lewiston.

Benson Lossing
Pictorial Field Book of the War of 1812
Chapter XXVIII, 1869

When Murray had gained full possession of the fort, he fired one of its largest cannon as a signal of success for the ear of General Riall, who, with a detachment of British regulars and about five hundred Indians, was waiting for it at Queenston.

Riall immediately put his forces in motion, and at dawn crossed the Niagara to Lewiston, and took possession of the village without much opposition from Major Bennett and a detachment of militia who were stationed on Lewiston Heights at Fort Grey. At the same time a part of Murray's corps plundered and destroyed the little village of Youngstown (only six or eight houses), near Fort Niagara.

Full license was given by Riall to his Indian allies, and Lewiston was sacked, plundered, and destroyed -- made a perfect desolation. This accomplished, the invaders pushed on toward the little hamlet of Manchester (now Niagara Falls Village); but, when ascending Lewiston Heights, they were met and temporarily checked and driven back by the gallant Major Mallory, who, with forty Canadian volunteers, came down from Schlosser and fought the foe for two days as they pushed him steadily back toward Buffalo. He could do but little to stay the march of the desolator.

The whole Niagara frontier on the American side, from Fort Niagara to Tonawanda Creek, a distance of thirty-six miles, and far into the interior, was swept with the besom of destruction placed by British authority in the hands of savage pagans. Manchester, Schlosser, and Tuscarora Village shared the fate of Youngstown and Lewiston.

Free course was given to the bloodthirsty Indians, and many innocent persons were butchered, and survivors were made to fly in terror through the deep snow to some forest shelter or remote cabin of a settler far beyond the invaders' track.

Buffalo, too, would have been plundered and destroyed had not the progress of the foe been checked by the timely destruction of the bridge over the Tonawanda Creek.

But the respite for doomed Buffalo was short. Riall and his followers returned to Lewiston, crossed over to Queenston, and on the morning of the 28th appeared at Chippewa, under the command of Lieutenant General Drummond.

In the meantime the alarm had spread over Western New York, and the inhabitants were thoroughly aroused. General McClure had sent out a stirring address to the "Inhabitants of Niagara, Genesee, and Chautauqua," urging them to repair immediately to Lewiston, Schlosser, and Buffalo.[1]

---

[1] U.S. General McClure's Address can be found in Cruikshank's Documentary History of the Campaigns, 1908. The address is dated Dec. 18, 1813, the day before the attack on Lewiston. He warns Western New York residents of an impending attack and states that Canadian men are being forced into service. "Every man in the province is required to take up arms and he that refuses is inhumanely butchered." He states, "Six or eight of their most respected inhabitants (Canadians) have fallen victim to their barbarity."

Desperately seeking manpower and volunteers, McClure further states, "I have received intelligence from a credible inhabitant of Canada (who has just escaped from thence) that the enemy are concentrating all their forces and boats at Fort George and have fixed upon tomorrow night for attacking Fort Niagara -- and should they succeed they will lay waste to our whole frontier... All who have arms and accoutrements will do well to bring them; and all who have horses will come mounted."

It is evident that McClure thought that the British attack was planned for the following night, the 19th. However, the attack began the night of the 18th, the same day McClure penned his address, which would indicate that there was little time for the intelligence to reach Fort Niagara, let alone the residents. At approximately 10pm, on Dec. 18, 1813, the British began crossing the Lower Niagara River and landing near today's Stella Niagara. The British were able to storm through Fort Niagara's front gate, in the early morning hours of the 19th, without firing a shot in the nighttime raid. Lewiston, for all practical purposes, was left defenseless.

Fortress Niagara
The Newsletter-Journal of the Old Fort Niagara Association
June 2002, by Harry DeBan
(Source: Canadian Archives)

Statement from U.S Gen. McClure to the citizens of Canada several weeks before the British Canadians retook Ft. George.

Address To the Inhabitants of the Upper Province of CANADA:
Brig. General McClure, Commanding on the Niagara Frontier, finds the Upper Province deserted by the British Army and abandoned by its Government...

In the peculiar situation of the inhabitants, it is essential to their security that some regulation should be established for their government, while the American Army has the power to enforce them. The General regrets to say, that illegal, unauthorized and forbidden pillage has been committed by a few, who are lost to all honor and insensible of the obligations of a soldier. To arrest such practices, to afford all the protection in his power, and to ensure safety to the property and persons of the inhabitants who are now under his control, the General has issued this address...

The employment of the Indians has been a source of extreme regret to the General. But, finding them called out by the government of The United States, and expecting to attack a British Army who has long employed them in scenes of atrocity and outrage at which humanity shudders, he was driven to the only alternative left him of using the same weapon against our enemies which they had used against ourselves.

That the British Army had abandoned their encampments and fled before the American force, does not weaken the necessity which he was under, of employing the Indians before he knew the enemy had absconded. At the same time, it is due to them to say, that the American Indians have conducted themselves far better than could have been expected, if the example of the British officers, and British savages be a criterion.

Not a single individual has been scalped or tomahawked by them... No Prisoner of War has been Burnt, the Dead are not thrown into the Public highways, Women and Children have not been massacred... nor has private property been destroyed, except in cases where the former conduct of the owners required exemplary retaliation. The property which they have plundered, has in cases where it was possible been restored to the inhabitants at the expense of The United States; and when the necessity of their employment ceased to exist, the Indians were sent to the American side of the Niagara River, beyond the reach of temptation, to wait until circumstances justified another call upon them.

To insure that forbearance, the inhabitants have an easy duty to perform... Let Them Be Perfectly Neutral, let them abstain from communication with the British Army and remain at home quietly pursuing their avocations. Those who conduct differently will incur the penalties of vigorous Martial Law! The character of our free republican government and the nature of out institutions, will justify your expectation of security and protection. All civil magistrates will continue to exercise functions of their offices merely as conservators of the Peace; as far as they are able, they will preserve order and quiet among the inhabitants. The existing laws of the Province, so far as they regard the Public Peace. and not interfering with the regulations of the Army, will be considered in force until other measures are taken.

The Magistrates are particularly required to give information at Head Quarters of all violence's committed by American Troops on citizens, unless they are authorized by a written order. The General enjoins the inhabitants to submit to their Magistrates, and those who refuse obedience will be reported to Head Quarters.

The Brig. General invites all the inhabitants who are disposed to be peaceable, orderly, and neutral, to return to their homes and business. He cannot promise complete security, but he engages as far as his power extends, to protect the innocent, the unfortunate, and the distressed.

Geo. McClure
Commanding Niagara Frontier
Head Quarters, Fort George, October 16, 1813

J. Boardman Scovell
History of the Niagara Portage
Published by Lewiston-Queenston Rotary Club
Copyright 1949, 1951

Some years ago when the Cibola burned at its wharf here, it was feared that the fire would be communicated to the warehouse on the wharf and so to the old custom house in the basement of the old American Hotel, which actually happened. But before it occurred, a group of young men moved all of the contents of the custom house across Water Street to the New York Central Station.

All of the papers were sorted, among which was found the account book of Jonas Harrison who, as heretofore stated, was the first Collector of Customs and the first Collector of Internal Revenue in this district. In the account book, which is now in the library of the Buffalo Historical Society, was found a copy of his accounts for the then current year and of his letter of transmission to the Secretary of the Treasury, written here four days after the burning of this village.

It can be considered to be true as it was written in his official capacity as Collector and as he was a member of the Harrison family which has given two presidents to the United States. In it he tells of his escape to Batavia, mentions that he and his family have nothing in the world except the clothes which they were wearing and the vacant lot on which their residence with its contents stood, and suggests promptness in remitting his semi-annual salary to become due on December 31st.

In the letter he also tells of the conditions in Lewiston, saying, "Every house in the village, save one, has been burned; and the bodies of the massacred lie about the streets, all of them scalped, many of them disemboweled, some with their tongues cut out, and all of them now being eaten by the hogs."

The movies "Drums along the Mohawk" and "Northwest Passage" were not over drawn. Do not say or think, "It could not happen here," for it did happen here and even worse than portrayed in the movies.

Helen B. Kimball
A Homely Approach to Lewiston, NY 1800-1954
Niagara County Historical Society, 1954

What was left from the burning of Lewiston? Mr. J. B. Scovell in his history of the Niagara Portage quotes the records of Jonas Harrison, first Collector of Customs, "Every house in the village, save one, has been burned." That is identified by Mr. Scovell as the tavern of the Hustler's on the northeast corner of Center and 8th Street.

The other building mentioned in early writings is the log stable belonging to Solomon Gillette. We can accept that because Jonas Harrison says "house" and he probably wouldn't have mentioned a log stable in his report to the government. Solomon lived first in a log hut near the present water tower, and then later near Hibbard's service station.[1] Log stables could have been in either place, who knows?

The present residents of the village who have passed the age of seventy years say that a house formerly standing on the corner of 6th and Center and occupied for many years by Michael Burke, the village builder, was always known as the "House Left Standing." Mrs. Lucy Williams Hawes, writing in 1887 of Lewiston, whose little book is quoted in some of the legal documents pertaining to the village property, says that the "House Left Standing" had disappeared.

Some enterprising person in 1900 issued a mailing folder of pictures of Lewiston. Included is a picture of an old house on the lot directly east of the Frontier House, the caption of which reads, "Only house left standing..." As the caption under several of the other pictures are slightly erroneous as to dates, we question this one.

---

[1] The water tower was located at the base of the Escarpment, in line with Portage Road, very near where the tree with the white cross is located today. Hibbard's service station was located where the Hibbard's liquor store and custard stand are currently located near Center St. and Portage Road.

So as you walk through the village of Lewiston and try to identify the house which was spared, some one is sure to point out the last mentioned. That story has been current for fifty years. As for me, I'll settle for the Hustler's Tavern. The Sage place is surely a survival but that is beyond the boundary of Jonas Harrison's report.

The hardy settlers, returned in the spring of 1814 and began rebuilding their homes, they were joined by several more in 1815 and the expansion of Lewiston really began in earnest. It is from that year that the oldest standing houses really date, the ones we see as we walk down Center Street.

Miscellaneous References

Reminiscences of Niagara
Published by William Pool, 1872.

In June 1812, on the declaration of war between the United States and Great Britain, most of the inhabitants removed to the interior, but generally returned and remained until December 1813; when the British and their Indian allies invaded and laid waste our defenseless frontier. Buildings and property of every description were destroyed; many unresisting persons were killed; and others only escaping with their lives, were in some cases reduced to extreme want and suffering. Nothing was saved, except two or three small dwellings and the log tavern, set on fire, but extinguished by persons at hand, after the hasty departure of the enemy. No buildings were again erected until after the close of the war, in 1815.

Diary of Charles Askin, Canadian Militia
Documentary History of the Campaign Upon the Niagara
Frontier in 1812-14, Cruikshank, Vol. IX, 1908

Just as the first boat load of Indians had reached the other (American) shore, the news of the fort (Ft. Niagara) being taken reached them. They immediately pushed off for Lewiston, and General Riall with the Royals and 41st marched to the same place. There were about sixty artillery at that place, who took to their heels as soon as they heard the yells of the Indians. About 12 or 13 of the enemy were killed at Lewiston, several of them inhabitants of the place.

Unfortunately, there was liquor in most of the houses, and, not withstanding the exertions of the officers of the Indian Department, the Indians soon got intoxicated and were outrageous. Several men of the regular troops got drunk also. The Indians plundered the houses, and then set fire to them. We were obliged to keep a strong guard over the poor inhabitants -- men, women and children -- to prevent them from being killed by the Indians. Indeed, Indians got so drunk that they did not know what they were about; two of their own Indians were killed by them and one of the 41st Regiment. Mr. Caldwell was shot through the thigh by one of them and young McDougall has his arm broke by another, who struck him with a tomahawk.

Indians, regulars, militia were plundering everything they could get hold of. Immense quantities of things were brought over from Lewiston to Queenston. At Youngstown, there were one or more stores from which everything was taken by the plunderers. I never witnessed such a scene before and hope I shall not again.

LIST OF SUFFERERS ON THE NIAGARA FRONTIER
(Lewiston, Youngstown, Above the Escarpment, and on Ridge Road to Lockport.)

This list is among papers that have been preserved by the Buffalo Historical Society[1] entitled, "List of Sufferers on the Niagara Frontier" without date or signature. The list is obviously incomplete but gives a description of the circumstances various citizens found themselves confronting. This is partial list, including sections of Niagara Falls not listed. This is a reprint of the list as published in Louis Babcock's The War of 1812 on the Niagara Frontier, published in 1927.

Lewiston

Benjamin Barton: House and office at Lewiston burnt, large barn on farm, not in want.

Hugh Howel. Innkeeper: hired house burnt, presumed not to have lost much; not in want; in Ontario.

John R. Smith. Innkeeper; house, shed, etc, burnt; himself and family said to be at large in Canada where he formerly lived.

Joshua Fairbanks. Merchant. House, etc. in Lewiston burnt; farm house and barn, with a large quantity of wheat, together with still house and still on the road to Schlosser all destroyed; not in want.

Townsend Bronson & Co. Merchants; storehouse, farm house and barn burnt; not in want.

Mrs. Mariamne Alvord. House and barn burnt; husband killed; herself with four small children in Ontario with Aaron Vanorman, her brother in law; worthy woman and must be in urgent want.

---

[1] Louis Babcock, The War of 1812 on the Niagara Frontier, 1927

Jonas Harrison. House and barn burnt; not in want.

Thomas Slayton. Hired house burnt; supposed not to have lost anything.

Dr. William Smith. Office, etc. destroyed; not in want.

Thomas Hustler. Innkeeper; house, barn and shed burnt; not in want.

Solomon Gillette. House etc. burnt; himself a prisoner; two sons killed; helpless wife with three small children, now between Batavia and Ridge Road; in distress; objects of prudent charity.

Mrs. Lewis. Husband, Reuben Lewis, killed; herself with four small children supposed to be near Aurora in Cayuga and as poor as can be conceived; objects of prudent charity.

Youngstown

Mrs. Agnes Greensitt. Her husband died last summer, leaving her and six or seven children; her house and furniture destroyed by the enemy on the 19th of December last; supposed to be with her children in Ontario County; presumed to be in want.

Elijah Hatheway. Lost a small log house and stable; residence unknown, presumed not to be in want.

John McBride. On the River Road towards Lewiston; house and furniture destroyed; wife and two or three children; supposed to be in Ontario County and probably in want; himself a prisoner with the enemy.

Isaac Swain. House, etc, destroyed; himself and family in Genesee County; not in want.

Jabez Hull. Hire house burnt; furniture, etc., destroyed; family in Ontario County; himself a prisoner; from circumstances presumed not to be in present want.

William Arbuthnot, William McBride, Alexander McBride. The two former prisoners, the latter with his family in Niagara County. They were tanners; their home, barn and tannery at first not burnt, since reported to have been; not in want.

Alexander Millar. Farmer; house, barn, etc, burnt; himself taken prisoner, since liberated and son still a prisoner; himself and family in Ontario; rich - large funds in different banks, besides abundant other property.

From the Top of the Mountain (Escarpment) to Manchester (now Niagara Falls, NY)

Abiather Buck. Himself a prisoner; wife and child on the road for Ontario; no property; objects of prudent charity.

Joseph Hewitt. Home and barn burnt; not in want.

Mrs. March. Hired house burnt; husband killed; herself and family on the way to Ontario; poor; objects of prudent charity.

Isaac Colt. Innkeeper; house, shed and barn burnt; not in want.

Henry Brother. Himself absent; family in Ontario and in want.

Benjamin Hopkins. Hired house burnt and with it his whole property destroyed; himself and wife in a bad state of health; two small children; in Seneca County, in urgent want.

Silas Hopkins. Home and barn burnt; not in want.

Ephraim Hopkins. Hired house burnt; supposed to have lost nothing; not in want.

Dr. Park. Elderly infirm man; large family; house and barn burnt; himself and family now live in Newtown; supposed to be in urgent want.

James Murray. Hired house burnt; wife and small family in Utica, himself in Niagara County; supposed to be in want.

Jacob Hovey. Small family; house, etc. burnt; carpenter and also...

Ebenezer Hovey. House etc. burnt; also carpenter; both with their families supposed to be in Canandaigua; present circumstances not actually known; worthy men.

Gad Pierce. Home etc. burnt; large family in Genesee County; not in want.

From Hustler's[1] at Lewiston to Widow Forsyth's[2], now Warren's on the Ridge Road

Mrs. Gardner. House and barn burnt, husband killed; saved some of her property, but presumed to be in want; herself with three or four children in Ontario.

John Beach. House and barn burnt; not in want; family in Ontario.

Lemuel Cooke. House etc. burnt; not in want; at Geneseo.

Lothrop Cooke. Lived in house with his father; had been some time sick and had his leg amputated; not well when the Indians came over; wife out of health; they have three small children; very poor; now at Geneseo, Ontario County.

---

[1] Hustler's Tavern was located on the Northeast corner of Center and 8th Streets in the Village of Lewiston.

[2] Vernette Genter, former Town of Cambria Historian, The Evolution of Niagara County. "Joseph Forsyth and his wife, Mary Ganson Forsyth, came to Cambria in 1805, and in 1806 opened a tavern in a log house at the east end of the Niagara Road. John replaced the cabin with a clapboard house in 1809 and operated the tavern there. He died in 1812, leaving his wife and four small children alone to face the dangers not only in the country, but of war as well. Mrs. Forsyth had continued to operate the tavern after her husband's death, and it was here that Ezra Warren, a soldier and native of Vermont, was stationed during the war to arrest deserters. After his discharge, he returned to Vermont, but unable to forget the widow Forsyth, he returned to Cambria to marry her. He became a prominent citizen of the area and proprietor of the tavern. Warrens Corners is named for him (Rt. 270 & 104). The former tavern has been, for many years, the home of the Floyd Yousey family. Mrs. Forsyth Warren rests in the family cemetery located on a knoll behind the house, between her two husbands and surrounded by the graves of their family members."

Ezra St. John. House burnt and all his property destroyed; himself and family taken prisoners; since returned without anything; now in Semphronius, Cayuga County; in want.

Hugh A. Wilson. House burnt and all his property destroyed, now in Ontario; in want.

John Groves. Hired house burnt; all his property destroyed; now in Ontario County; in want.

William Miller. Log house burnt; not in want.

_____Pitcher. Hired house burnt; family taken prisoner; not in want; in Onondaga County.

James Latta and son, John Latta. House and shop burnt. Now in Geneva; not in want.

William Molyneux. Barn burnt, some property destroyed, family in Genesee County; not in want.

Rev. Andrew Gray. House burnt; family in Geneseo; not in want.

John Robinson. House burnt; together with the destruction of all his property; himself and large young family at Geneseo, in want.

Rufus Spalding. House burnt, property destroyed, but not in want.

Mrs. Totten. House burnt; in Niagara County; not in want.

_____ Southard. All his property plundered and destroyed; himself and family now in Avon, Ontario County, in low state of poverty.

William Bartholomew. Loss very trifling; not in want.

Ray Marsh. Loss not great, but now poor; in Genesee County, presumed to be in want.

_____ Omstead. House burnt; family in Genesee; poor and in want.

Charles Redman (Redmond?). Hired house burnt, all property destroyed; family on the Ridge Road, in want.

Solomon Gould. House burnt; presumed to be in want; in Bloomfield.

David Jones. Lost some property, not in want.

Aaron Childs. House burnt; family in Ontario; not in want.

Cushman Smith. Presumed rather to have gained than lost; not in want.

Ely Harris. Loss nothing; not in want.

Jonathan Fasset. One of the speculators; not in want.

Solomon Hersey. Loss trifling; not in want.

Polly Hopkins. Widow, since married; loss trifling; not in want.

Elijah Newton. Speculator; not in want, as presumed.

Lewis Hawley. Speculator; not in want, as presumed.

_____ Glines. Speculator; presumed not to be in want.

_____ Warren. House burnt; property all destroyed; family in Ontario, presumed to be in want.

Akish Pool. House burned; family in Ontario; presumed to be in want.

Daniel Howel. Loss nothing; not in want.

Isaac B. Tyler. Speculator; presumed not to be in want.

James Clark. Loss nothing; now with his family in Ontario; poor and presumed to be in want.

_____ Babcock. Loss trifling; self and family in Ontario; poor and presumed to be in want.

Loring Doney. Blacksmith; loss trifling; self and family now in Ontario County; poor and presumed to be in want.

William Howel. Loss considerable; not in want.

Elnathan Holmes. Speculator; presumed not to be in want.

Aaron Beach. Speculator; presumed not to be in want.

_____ Neil. Loss nothing; remained the whole time at home, without the limits assigned to themselves by the enemy.

Alex. Allen. Loss nothing; but poor and presumed to be in want; residence unknown.

Names of Known Americans Killed
During the British Attack
Lewiston, New York
December 19, 1813

Whatever local population records existed were destroyed in the attack. This information is very sketchy, and the exact names and number of people killed will never be known.

Helen Mead
Dr. Joseph Alvord
Jervis Gillette, age 7
Thomas Marsh
Frink (or Finch)
Tiffany
Dr. Molly[2]
Mr. Trowbridge

Mead, the teamster
Miles Gillette, age 19
Pitcher Family[1]
John Marsh
William Gardner
Reuben Lewis
Mr. Mack

Members of Militia:
Captain Rose
Lt. John M. Lowe
George W. Jones, son of Horatio Jones
James W. Jones, son of Horatio Jones

---

[1] Mentioned as killed in the Geneva Gazette, Jan. 5, 1814. However, the family's name is included on the "List of Sufferers" as taken prisoner and then later living in Onondaga County.

[2] Dr. Molly was "a practitioner at the Eleven Mile Creek (Wilson, NY) of humane and amiable character, and had gone to Lewiston merely as an act of benevolence to render medical aid... he entreated them (the British) to save his life...and one of them ran a bayonet through his abdomen, and as he drew it out, his bowels followed. The good man placed his hand on his own bowels, and walked 6 miles to Ft. Niagara and in 15 minutes bid a final adieu to this wicked world." Niles Weekly Register, Dec. 24, 1814.

Names of Known Tuscarora Men Who
Defended Lewiston During the British Attack
December 19, 1813

Solomon Longboard, Sachem[1,3]
Longboard's two sons[1]
Isaac Allen[1,4]
William Alvis[2]
Jim Basket[2]
John Beach[2,4]
Big-Fish[2]
Blacksnake[2]
Black Chief[1]
John Black Nose[1]
Peter Black Nose[4]
David Cusick[1]
George Cusick[2]
John Cusick[1]
Joseph Cusick[1,2,4]
Gau-ya-re-na-twa[1]
Litte Fish[2]
John Fox[2,4]
John Green[1]
Isaac Green[1,4]
Surgin Green[1]
Isaac Grouse (Crouse)[2]
Sgt. Grouse (Crouse)[2]
John Henry[2]
Col. Aaron Johnson[2,3]
Washington Lewis[2]

Littlegreen[3]
Seth Lyon[2]
Isaac Miller[2,4]
John Mt. Pleasant[1,4]
John Obediah[1]
Ovid[3]
Adam Patterson[2,4]
Harry Patterson[1]
John Patterson[2,4]
Aaron Pembleton[1,4]
James Pembleton[1]
Samuel Pembleton[2]
"Little Billy" Printup[1,2,4]
George Printup[1,2,4]
John Printup[1,2]
William Printup[1,2,4]
Thomas Smith[2]
Peter Sky[4]
Jacob "Col. Jacobs" Taylor[1]
Isaac Thompson[2]
Samuel Thompson[1,4]
John Tobacco[2]
Capt. Williams[1]
Henry Williams[2,4]

Sources
1 Chief Elias Johnson, History of the Tuscaroras, 1881
2 Toni Jollay Prevost, Indians from New York, Vol. 3., 1995
3 Chipman Turner, Dark Days on the Frontier, 1879
4 Index of Awards, Soldiers of the War of 1812, Albany, 1860

Source	Number of Lewiston civilians killed	Lewiston civilian names mentioned as killed	Number of Tuscarora Heroes
Chipman P. Turner, Dark Days on the Frontier, 1879	46	Dr. Alvord, Miles Gillette, Gillette boy, William Gardner (scalped and decapitated), Jones' brothers, Helen Mead, Mead, Thomas Marsh, Tiffany, Finch, John Marsh, Frink	
Clara L. Sisson Williams, An Experience of 1813, Recalling Pioneer Days, 1922 (granddaughter of Solomon Gillette)	"Eight or 10 were killed or scalped, with the exception of one, whose head was cut off."	Miles Gillette, age 19, and his step-brother, Jervis Gillette, age 7	
Cruikshank, Drummond's 1813 Winter Campaign	Some		47
Orsamus Turner, Pioneer History of the Holland Lane Purchase, 1850		Dr. Alvord, Miles Gillette and a younger brother, sons of the early pioneer Solomon Gillette, Thomas Marsh, William Gardner, Tiffany, Finch.	"a small band"
Unknown American officer, letter to the Albany Argus, Dec. 26, 1813	"It is not yet ascertained how many were killed as most of the bodies were thrown into the burning houses and consumed."	William Gardner, Deputy Sheriff, John M. Low, Ezra St. John*, Attorneys, Dr. Alvord, and "six others whose names I've forgotten." *later reported alive.	

Source	Number of Lewiston civilians killed	Lewiston civilian names mentioned as killed	Number of Tuscarora Heroes
Elias Johnson, Legends, Traditions of the Iroquois, 1888			35
Joshua Cooke, The Pioneer Association of Niagara County, Reminiscences of Lewiston, 1902	"nearly a dozen were shot down"	Dr. Alvord. "He was a cripple, and, attempting to escape on horseback, was shot down and tomahawked. When he was found his poor fingers were slit down to the wrists with the hatchets, as he had vainly held them up to parry the blows or to ask for mercy.	"a little band"
History of Lewiston, NY, Landmarks of Niagara County, William Pool, 1897	"about twelve"	Dr. Alvord, Thomas Marsh, Jervis Gillette, Tiffany, Finch, Reuben Lewis (who "agreed with a neighbor that he would never be taken alive, he fought after he was wounded until the enemy came up and killed him.")	

Isaac C. Cooke

Transcription of Handwritten Letter from Isaac C. Cooke, eyewitness to the British Attack on Lewiston. A copy of this letter was discovered in September 2010, and was added to this book as part of the third edition. Transcription by Jeanne Cooke Collins, Denver CO, October 6, 2010. Jeanne is a descendant of Isaac Cooke, who was the son of Lemuel, and brother to Lothrop and Bates. The location or existence of the original letter is unknown. Original copy on legal size, 3 pages. Original paragraphing, spelling/misspelling, punctuation, and capitalization retained.

The nineteenth day of December 1813 was to the residents of Lewiston and Niagara Frontier a Memorable day, long to be remembered by those who escaped from the Tomahawk and Scalping knife of the British Savages. The british came over and took Fort Niagara, without resistace, murdering the Sick and disabled as well as the hale, at the same time a force of some three hundred Britsh and Moha__ came over Crossi^{n}g at the 3 mile meadow (now Hotchkis farm) and on hearing the british salute fired at the Fort, started like blood-hounds, for Lewiston, where they took the Guard by surprise killing some, (Miles Gittel) and making prisoners of the others This caused a general stampede, Dr. Alvord in attempting to escape was shot by the Indians and butchered. They took the Gittel family prisoners and along about (where Powell now lives) killed a little boy (six or seven) and scalped him, Our women folks started off on foot, Mother, Laura, Amelia, ~~Amanda~~, your mother and Children, Lewis, Samuel, the Baby Bates (I think about one month old) Father, and Isaac, got the ox teams to the door, and a few things were thrown on, Bates took Lothrop in his arms and put him on the sleigh, his leg had then been amputated only 2 weeks, Father drove the sleigh on which was the invalid, and Bates the other, after us came the british hell-hounds, at the west corner of our orchard they butchered a poor fellow named Tiffany, and a little east of Hulls they killed another Majr Wm Gardner, on they came, five on horses, overtaking us at place where the Indian road enterred the Ridge Road as the Indians came up with us they called out. <u>Stop, Stop</u>. Fathers team ran against a log, and stopped, one rode around the sleigh, stricking a full blow with a sword at Lothrops head, but his horse jumped and he missed him, the sword striking a brass kettle. Bates had caught a gun from his sleigh, and running north about four rods, took aim at one of them as he sat on his horse, fired and shot him through the neck. Lothrop said to Father, Bates has killed that Indian he came down head foremost, at that instant, two of the Indians fired at Bates with Rifles, missing him, he then ran down the hill coming to me, (Isaac) A party Tuscaroras going up the Indian hill, hearing the firing on the road below wheeled about, firing and whooping, which freighend the British Indians, two of them catching hold of the one that was shot in the neck ran back, leaving him dead about in front of the the Maj Lgon place After they left, Father called to Bates to come back, we started the teams going as fast as we could fearing the Indians would overtake us again, they did come nearly as far as Old Bill Howells and seeing there several men with arms they retired, the women and children by riding and walking, got as far as Forsyth's (now Warren's Corners) When we came up with them, they having been told that the Indians overtook us and we were all murdered, which would have been the case, had it not been for the fortunate circumstance of the Tuscaroras being there just at that particular time.

When we met at Forsyths, it was indeed a happy family meeting, especially to the women and children who had in consequence of reports of our Masscre given up all hopes of ever seeing us again There being no time spare, (now about dusk) we started east, through the <u>Eleven Mile-Woods</u> arriving half-way at a log House, (Brewer's) at about 8 OClock P. M. here we halted for the night, in a room about 11 by 18, took Lothrop in, making a place in one corner, there were about twenty in that room besides ourselves, two women, and several children that had come through the woods from Fort Niagara; well as soon as possible Mother got an iron pot, (we had 3 quarters of beef and two bags of flour in our sleigh) in which she fried the meat, baked a cake in the ashes, cleaned out the iron pot made tea in it, and we had a general feast. The next day made seven miles.

Lothrop suffered much pain with his leg and great deal with a sore on the small of his back occasioned by constantly laying on his back   We had a tedious journey of three days to Geneseo, (the home of the Wadsworths) where we found true and generous friends

written by father, Emily

The Indian killed by Bates was an Ottawa brave.
foot note by E. M. Cooke

IN APPRECIATION

Thank you to Neil Patterson, Sr., his wife Francene, of the Tuscaror⁓ Nation, and Suzanne Dietz from the Town of Porter, and Patrick Kavanagh from Buffalo, for their valued input.

Thank you to Pam Hauth, the director of the Historical Association and Lewiston Museum, and volunteer, MaryAlice Eckert, who helped collect and transcribe much the material in this book.

Thank you to Lewiston-Porter art teacher and Historical Association volunteer, Cindy Sanchez, for the cover art.

I must also mention the Herculean job that was accomplished by Canadian Lt. Col. E. Cruikshank in 1908 when he collected and edited The Documentary History of the Campaigns Upon the Niagara Frontier for the Lundy Lane's Historical Society. This compilation of material includes all of the written correspondence and published articles pertaining to the War of 1812, in chronological order, from both sides of the conflict. It was a remarkable feat that has awed students of the War ever since and made the study of the War much easier and dramatically more insightful. Thank you, Col. Cruikshank!

About the Author

Lee Simonson has been a resident of Lewiston, NY, for 50 years. After serving as a Niagara County Legislator for over three decades, he became a volunteer for the Historical Association of Lewiston. He was the project director for the Freedom Crossing Monument, and is now the director for the proposed Tuscarora Heroes Monument to be unveiled December 19, 2013. He is an independent small businessman and he and his wife, Brenda, have two grown children, Jill and Robin.

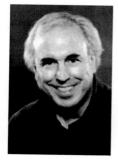

THANK YOU FOR YOUR SUPPORT

The Historical Association of Lewiston, Inc., wishes to express its
gratitude to the board members of the Village and Town of
Lewiston for their past and future support.
Current board members as of August 2012:

Town of Lewiston
Steven Reiter, Supervisor
Alfonso Bax   Ernest Palmer
Michael Marra   Ronald Winkley

Village of Lewiston
Terry Collesano, Mayor
Bruce Sutherland   Victor Eydt
Nicholas Conde   Dennis Brochey

Historical Association of Lewiston Board of Trustees
Bruce Sutherland, President
Leandra Collesano, Vice President
Steven Frey, Treasurer
Timothy Tutko, Secretary
Ellen Augello   Claudia Carnes   Zach Collister
Victor Eydt   Michael Marra   Tricia Mezhir
Lisa Ohanessian   Edward Perlman   Robert Welch

Director: Pam Hauth

And a special thank you to all of the Historical Association
volunteers and members who help preserve and
promote Lewiston's rich heritage.